The

B I

The Hair
BIBLE

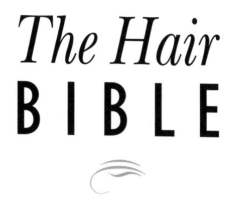

A Complete Guide to
Health and Care

PHILIP KINGSLEY

AURUM PRESS

OCT 2 2003

First published in Great Britain
2003 by Aurum Press Ltd
25 Bedford Avenue, London WC1B 3AT

Copyright © 2003 Philip Kingsley

Design by M Rules

A catalogue record for this book is available from the
British Library.

ISBN 1 85410 906 5

1 3 5 7 9 10 8 6 4 2
2003 2005 2007 2006 2004

Printed in Great Britain by MPG Books Ltd, Bodmin

Contents

Acknowledgements

Writing this book has made me realize, yet again, how lucky I am to have such a wide range of expert friends from whom I have been able to seek information and advice. Also, how incredibly lucky I am to have a team of trichologists and staff who go beyond the call of duty. I particularly want to single out Claire Edgecombe, my irreplaceable personal assistant, who has worked all hours with my numerous and interminable (it seems) re-writes in the attempt to make my deadline, as well as smoothing out my life.

Others I am indebted to include Glenn Lyons, my London Clinical Director; Brian Thompson, my New York Clinic Research Director; Carole Michaelides, who runs my clinic at Harrods; and Michael Steinberg, who, similar to Claire Edgecombe in London, smoothes my life in New York.

My professional advisory friends include Walter Futterweit MD, Clinical Professor of Medicine, Division of Endocrinology, Mount Sinai Hospital, New York City; Jeffrey I. Mechanick MD (Associated Clinical Professor) and his associate Elise Brett MD; Walter Unger MD (Toronto and New York); Jeremy Gilkes MD, FRCP; and Professor Stephen Franks MD Hon MD FRCP FRCOG, Imperial College, Institute of Reproductive and Development Biology, Hammersmith Hospital, London.

The list would not be complete without thanking Marcelle d'Argy Smith (who wrote the foreword to my last book) for her encouragement; Caron Banfield for her spectacular front-cover styling; Terry O'Neill for painstakingly photographing it; and to Piers Burnett at Aurum Press for his ideas and guidance.

Last, but by no means least, my wife Joan and my daughters Katherine, Anabel, Susan and Helen, who have helped in so many ways with remarks and choosing a suitable title for this book.

I am dedicating this book to Joan, who has put up with me for so many years!

Introduction

When my publisher, Aurum Press, told me that *Hair: An Owner's Handbook* had sold out, I was surprised. I don't know why I should have been – my first book, *The Complete Hair Book* (Grosset and Dunlop USA, 1979), also sold out. It was reprinted in trade paperback for the USA and in a 'pocket' paperback by Magnum in the UK. All of them sold out. It was suggested that *Hair: An Owner's Handbook* was republished in paperback with a few updated changes. On reading it again, I realized that since 1995, its publication date, many things in the 'hair world' had changed, thus minor adjustments would not be sufficient to really bring it up-to-date.

In addition, I have been a regular weekly columnist for the *Sunday Times* for about three years. I write for their 'Style' magazine. At first I was asked to write a 'Hair tip of the week'. My tips got quite a following, and I was asked to do a series on the effects of hair colouring, in which I had half a column weekly for eight months. Now I have my own column called 'The Hair Doctor', in which I write about all aspects of scalp and hair. Another surprise was the subjects that seemed to have had the most impact – the largest response was an article on hair twiddling, that is, playing with and twisting your own hair. My clinic had 3600 responses, more than any other article before or since, so much so that I have written a chapter entitled 'Hair Twiddling' later in this book. Hair twiddling is much more common than thought, and it often results in a self-inflicted hair loss called Trichotillomania.

The past eight years have also seen the introduction of 'leave-in' conditioners as styling aids, more focus on hair protectors (particularly sun protection), another scare on the possible cancer-causing effects of hair colouring, and the plethora of new products. Hair transplantation is more sophisticated and can give results that were not possible eight years ago. There have been significant advances in hair loss, too, and these are discussed in detail together with yet another surprise, the incidence of PCOS (Polycystic Ovarian Syndrome) in women and its effect on hair thinning.

There is no doubt that hair loss, hair fall and hair thinning (not necessarily the same) remain the number one anxiety-causing problem. Their effect on quality of life is so far-reaching, the psychological impact so sadly underestimated, the myths so diverse and the management often so complicated (although usually successful). The disdain many doctors give it as being unimportant and not life-threatening but simply an issue of cosmetics and vanity has almost broken my heart when seeing young women disturbed, agitated and verging on suicide after being told to 'pull yourself together – you can always wear a wig' by their uncaring doctor.

It should be no surprise, therefore, that a lot of this book is given to the various forms and causes of hair loss. It will hopefully help to put your mind at rest and see the opportunities that are available. All the cosmetic aspects are discussed too: seasonal care, how to deal with dull hair, limp hair, frizzy hair, split ends, shampoos, conditioners, styling aids, colouring, perming, blow-drying, all the myths – in fact, everything you will ever need to know in your quest to attain the best and healthiest looking hair it is possible to have.

Hair – Sex and Psychology

You may wonder why you care about your hair so much. After all, if you were without it, you would still be alive – it doesn't hurt if you cut it. Yet how many times during the day do you look at your hair or touch it or think about it? *Why* does the way it looks, feels or behaves affect your morale so much? The answer is to do with sex.

It is impossible to understand the importance of human hair without appreciating its role as a sexual object. There is a vital link between sexuality and hair. To caress someone's hair, to fondle or play with it, even to smell it, is, consciously or not, a sexual act. How we style our hair, how it's cut, the care we give it and how we display it indicate to the world in a myriad of ways our sexual feelings, aggressions, insecurities, confidence or inhibitions. Hair is the single most important part of the anatomy affecting our psyche. We can wear the most fashionable clothes, the most expensive jewellery, our skin can be flawless but if our hair isn't right, we don't feel good. The reverse is also true.

Hair is a secondary sexual characteristic. The primary sexual characteristics are the genitals, but in virtually all cultures the human genitals are deliberately hidden from view. It is the taboo against genital display that gives hair much of its power as a sexual object. Hair is the only part of the human anatomy that can be sexually flaunted at will. The sexual nature of hair is so powerful that some societies demand its concealment or loss to symbolize sexual morality, celibacy or punishment. Nuns cut and then cover their hair, thus hiding their sexuality; Orthodox Jewish and Muslim women cover their hair in public as a sign of modesty; women collaborators in World War II had their heads shaved to desexualize as well as to punish them; monks shave the tops of their heads as a symbolic rejection of their sexuality. Labour camps in some countries shave not all of the head but only half to humiliate prisoners and make them figures of ridicule.

Female hair is seen as seductive and essentially sexual in meaning. The way in which hair has historically been categorized confirms the sexuality of hair. For instance, redheads have traditionally been thought of as wanton: in the Middle Ages they were seen as witches and charged with sexually luring men to make pacts with the Devil, who himself is pictured as red. Blondes are viewed as vulnerable, while dark-haired women are threatening. Women with long, lustrous hair send messages of sexual fertility, longing and availability. It is no coincidence that Lorelei and the mermaids, who in legends enticed men to their deaths, had long, free-flowing hair. Their sexual enticement was lethal. In the age-old mating game shiny, healthy-looking hair is seductive

The most popular female film stars, models and pop stars, past and present, have had long, loose hair: Betty Grable, Rita Hayworth, Marilyn Monroe, Kate Winslett, Britney Spears, Claudia Schiffer, Gwyneth Paltrow, Julia Roberts and Melanie Griffith, to name but a few. Long hair is thought of as being more feminine – softer and more sensual.

For men, hair is symbolic of virility and strength. This symbolism is so powerful that a Samson myth is common in most cultures. Great Samson lost his strength when Delilah cut his hair. In male primates hair displays are used to intimidate, to express fierceness, power and aggression. The same is true of human males. We commonly think of hairy men as being more virile, more commanding and dominant. Body hair, beards and moustaches contribute to this image of dominance and aggression. Traditionally, warriors have grown elaborate moustaches and beards, even when they know that beards offered an all-too-convenient handhold to the enemy. So important is hair as a symbol of masculine strength that some cultures created headdresses to exaggerate their virility and power. The bearskin helmets of the British Life Guards, the Indian chiefs' feather headdresses, the complicated headdresses of primitive tribes, the crowns of kings and emperors, the heroes' laurel wreaths – all are tokens of male power, potency and virility.

It is this symbolism that makes women in particular fear any damage to their hair. Thinning hair is connected with the loss of sexuality and femininity. The lack of body and lustre signifies failure to make oneself attractive. And hair thinning is associated with ageing – being less attractive and losing the ability to seduce.

In men, hair loss likewise represents loss of virility, masculinity and power – a symbolic castration. Take, for example, the American Indian practice of scalping enemies. They believed that once the scalp was removed, a man's strength was also gone and could not reinhabit his body. These scalps, which symbolized the enemy's stolen strength, were then worn as plaits by the Indians – the more scalps, the greater the warrior.

In many ways, hair, more than eyes, is the sexual mirror of the soul. In a covert way we love our hair. We long for it to be full and beautiful, and we cast covetous eyes on the hair of others. We use it to draw attention to ourselves, to attract and entice, to flaunt and seduce. It can make our day or ruin it, give elation or depression. We take more care of it, spend more time on it and nurture it more than any other part of our body. Our anxiety about it is often beyond belief. We can love it and caress it, loathe it and curse it, but the joy of good-looking, well-behaved hair framing your face gives a psychological boost second to no other.

2

Is Your Hair Dead or Alive?

Physiology Explained

I'm sure you've heard someone say that it doesn't matter what you do to your hair – it's dead anyway. But *is* it? No and yes. The hair outside your scalp, physiologically speaking, is dead. It has no blood, nerves or muscles. If cut, you feel no pain; nor does it bleed or pull a muscle when stretched. However, for a 'dead' fibre it is quite remarkable. A healthy hair will stretch up to 30 per cent of its length, can absorb its weight in water and can swell up to 20 per cent of its diameter. It has extraordinary insulating powers, rivalling that of asbestos. Its strength is greater than that of copper wire of the same diameter. An average head of hair can support 23 tons of weight. We change its colour, its shape, its curl, wash it, brush it, set it, spray it, tease it, pull it and rub it to an amazing degree, and yet despite all of this abuse, our hair can remain resilient and tough.

Hair is composed of *keratin*, a fibrous protein, and is built from cells not unlike those of the skin. The hair shaft consists of three layers: the outer *cuticle*, composed of overlapping cells, like fish scales or roof shingles; the *cortex*, comprising the hair's main bulk and colour; and the *medulla*, a thin core of transparent cells and air spaces. Hair grows from a single *follicle*, an indentation in the skin. Each of us is born with a specific number, which cannot be changed, and the size of the follicle determines the thickness of the hair. Some follicles have one hair, others may contain two or three. At the base of the follicle, lying in the dermis (the deeper layer of the skin), is the *papilla*, the bud of the hair where most growth takes place. Each follicle has its own blood, nerve and muscle supply. The nerves and the muscles give the hair its tactile properties, allowing the slightest movement to be felt. When the muscles contract, the hair stands up more and pinches the skin, causing 'goose bumps'. We inherit this characteristic from animals – the bristling quills of a porcupine and the hairs of a cat are exaggerated examples, as are the extremely sensitive whiskers of the cat family. The crinkling of sheep's wool is due to irregular contractions of the follicle muscles (called *arrector pili*) which change the shape of the follicle and, therefore, the characteristics of the wool produced. The blood capillaries surrounding the follicle carry the nourishment needed for cell production and growth. Again, hair is remarkable: its cell reproduction is the second most prolific of the human body, bone marrow being the first. This means that hair is extremely sensitive to changes going on within the body, and it is often as a result of these internal problems that hair loss can occur. But more about this in future chapters.

Hair grows about half an inch (1.25 centimetres) a month – faster in summer than in winter. The growth phase, or *anagen*, lasts an average of three to five years, so a full-length hair averages 18–30 inches. At the end of *anagen*, the hair enters *catagen*, a short intermediary phase prior to *telogen*, a resting phase when the hair is released and falls out. The follicle rests for three months, then the whole process is repeated. Each hair follicle is independent, having its own growth cycle at different times, otherwise all our hair would fall out at once! Instead, you lose only a certain number of hairs a day. The cycle can be disrupted by metabolic circumstances, the nature of which I shall explain later.

The average number of hairs on the human scalp is 120,000. Blondes tend to have more, redheads less. With 120,000 hairs and an average growth phase of four years, you can afford to lose 75–80 hairs a day. But it's not quite that simple – as you will see later in this book.

3

The Ethnic Behaviour of Hair

A further complication in the understanding of hair's physiology and behaviour patterns are the variations in ethnic hair types. Ethnic differences in hair are quite distinct. For example, Caucasians suffer the highest percentage of *male pattern hair loss,* Blacks have the second-highest incidence, while Orientals suffer the least. In American Indians male pattern hair loss is almost non-existent. On the other hand, Black women have the highest rate of *traction hair loss* (due to pulling and straightening), exceeding all other races combined. Caucasians are the only group with a large variation in hair colour, and there *is* an association between hair colour and baldness – the blonder the hair, the greater the susceptibility.

Evolutionary nuances together with nutritional and climate changes have all had their effect on human hair. In pre-human times an animal's coat colour, and the thickness and pattern of its fur, acted as a camouflage against enemies and protection against climate and sun. But human hair no longer has biological or protective functions: it is merely decorative. The shape, size and configuration of hair differ with each race, affecting handling and grooming requirements, although intermarriage does blur ethnic distinctions.

There are three basic ethnic groups, each having distinct hair characteristics. But there are also subgroups. For example, Caucasian hair can have a similar appearance to Black (African/American) hair, often called 'Afro' Hair, which is usually frizzy and fine (as discussed in the Black Hair section). This occurs mostly amongst Semitic races (Jewish and Arabic) who may be viewed as Afro-Asiatic anyway. An interesting feature in this sub-group is that males seem to be more prone to curly, frizzy hair than females – particularly at the sideburns.

Each hair type also has different shapes in cross-section, as shown in the photographs below.

BLACK HAIR

The hair shaft has a flat shape (see p.10) with a twisted configuration and a thin diameter. There are intermittent variations in diameter as the twisting occurs, which causes a recurrent weakening along each hair. Due to their curliness, the hairs wrap around

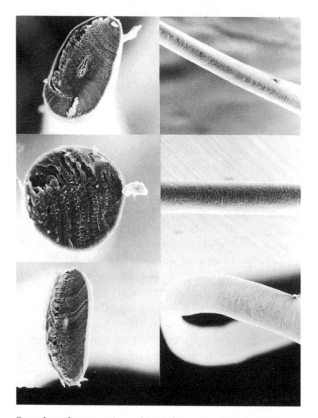

Strands and cross-sections of (top) Caucasian hair, (middle) Oriental hair and (bottom) Black hair

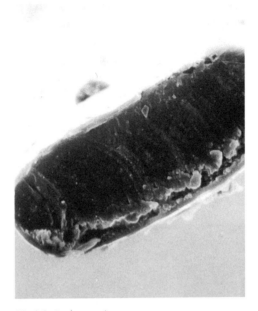

Black hair cross-section

each other, resulting in serious tangles; trying to de-tangle this type of hair can break it at its weak points, and the pulling may lead to stressing the hair follicles and traction hair loss. Because of the problems inherent in this type of hair, grooming presents a dilemma. Often there is an irresistible temptation to straighten tight, curly hair. Methods for straightening vary, but the most common are to set it on rollers and blow dry, hot comb or oil press it. None of these are exactly conducive to healthy hair and each invariably leads to traction hair loss and severe breakage.

The incidence and degree of traction loss in Black women are underestimated and often mistaken for other types of hair loss. It starts as a thinning at the front hairline, then receding continues with a general thinning all over, making this condition similar to male pattern hair loss. In another form, loss occurs all around the scalp edges, leaving what looks like an ill-fitting cap of hair. This type of thinning is called *banded traction alopecia*, because the hair loss is literally shaped like a band around the scalp.

Another type of traction hair loss is one in which hair comes out in clumps. The main causes of this 'patchy' hair loss are sleeping in rollers, wearing too tight braids (particularly in children) or, in adults, too tight rollers. This condition is not to be confused with alopecia areata, which is associated with psychological stress rather than the physical kind of traction stress.

Although I rarely recommend strong chemical procedures, I feel that rather than repeatedly subjecting the hair to these twisting and pulling traumas, it is better to use chemical hair straighteners. These work in the same way as a reverse perm: instead of using the solution to curl straight hair, it is used to straighten curly hair. On average this is done every twelve to sixteen weeks. There are obvious risks involved – more so than with a normal perm – because the chemical must be applied at scalp level to give the most successful effect. However, in the long term the benefits far outweigh the risks. Once the hair is straightened, none of the other procedures such as hot oil, pressing, pulling and hot combs are necessary. A further benefit is that chemically straightening hair encourages more frequent washing because the hair is easier to style. A common complaint amongst Black women who wash their hair too infrequently is the occurrence of an itchy scalp and flakiness. And contrary to popular thought, washing the hair frequently with the appropriate shampoos and conditioners makes hair less dry rather than more dry.

Colour

Hair is given its colour by the formation of *melanin* – pigment granules – in the hair follicle. Black hair is not necessarily truly black, but rather a combination of black and red pigment, giving shades from almost true black through to dark brown and auburn. Approximately 40 per cent of Black women have black to near-black hair, about 50 per cent have dark brown and 5–10 per cent have auburn shades. The use of hair-colouring products amongst Black females is thought to be quite high, increasing the risk of hair damage, especially when we consider the inherent variations in the diameter of the hairs and in styling methods. The most popular colours are the red shades, but blonde is becoming a close second and is potentially the most damaging (see Chapter 12 on 'Hair Colouring').

Care

The unique structure, processing, styling and grooming needs of Black hair make it the most vulnerable to damage, and frequent use of a specialized conditioner is mandatory. It is best to avoid the heavy, oily type of styling products, for although many are labelled 'oil free', they still leave an unpleasant coating to which dust and dirt cling, giving a dull greasy look instead of the shine they are meant to give.

Choice of product is often influenced by packaging, fragrance, colour and, of course, advertising. But a little knowledge of the purpose of the ingredients contained in a product will help you to choose more wisely. Chapter 29 on 'Formulations and Ingredients' will give you this information. However, as a general rule, when purchasing a conditioner look on the label for adjectives such as moisturizing, remoisturizing, emollient, deep conditioning, elasticizing, penetrative, intensive, or a combination of any of these.

Conditioners come in two categories – pre-shampoo and post-shampoo. With Black hair, both need to be used frequently. Rather than choose by trial and error, taking no notice of ingredients or claims, you should shop around carefully.

If you wish, you can try making your own treatment in the kitchen. A quite effective pre-shampoo deep conditioner can be made by whisking together the following ingredients in a blender:

2 eggs
2oz double cream
1oz castor oil
1oz melted unsalted butter
1oz purified water
Juice of ½ grapefruit

Refrigerate overnight if necessary and use as required. Apply the mixture to the whole length of the hair in sections. To distribute and penetrate, work into the hair with fingers or massage the scalp with a kneading motion for five to ten minutes and leave on for a further twenty minutes (or even overnight). Shampoo as usual with a remoisturizing shampoo and remoisturizing conditioner. Do this as often as possible until your hair is sufficiently improved. If you have a scalp or hair loss problem, apply the appropriate product to your scalp, followed by the above cream to your hair. Massage together. For some specific scalp treatments, see Chapter 8 on 'Hair Loss in Women' and Chapter 10 on 'Dandruff'. After rinsing the conditioner but before drying, apply a leave-in styling conditioner. There are many available and usually they have a descriptive word or phrase such as anti-frizz or frizz control. Chosen carefully, they can be very effective – particularly those containing various silicones (see p.157 on 'Silicones').

Limp Hair

A surprising number of Black women perceive their hair as 'limp'. It is not possible to have limp, curly hair, but there are reasons why it may be seen as such under certain circumstances. 'Limp' hair occurs only amongst Black women over twenty-five, and may become progressively noticeable. It is caused by repeated straightening procedures, which eventually reduce the hair's volume through traction loss. Also, straight hair appears to have less body and behaves 'limper' than wavy or curly hair. A double whammy, so to speak. Moreover, everyone over the age of forty begins to notice a diminished hair volume, a condition that may be confused with limpness.

Once hair has reached the stage of thinness at which it is perceived as limp, it may be too late to reverse the condition. Traction hair loss over a long duration is often irreversible. Age-induced thinning may also be irreversible unless discovered in its early stages and acted upon accordingly (see Chapters 8 and 22 on 'Hair Loss').

Treatment of limp hair is also discussed in the 'Hair Body' section (p.26). However, Black or any other type of very curly hair can be given more body by 'loose curling', a type of permanent wave that stops short of straightening but eases the tight curls into a looser, more manageable style.

CAUCASIAN HAIR

The individual Caucasian hair is oval in shape (see picture, p.14), mostly fine-textured and varying between straight and wavy. Approximately 70 per cent of Caucasians have fine-textured hair. This is the only ethnic group with large variations in hair colour – from white blond through to browns, reds and black. Of the two types of melanin (pigment) that give hair its colour, it is the blond/brown type that is predominant in Scandinavian and northern climates, whilst the blown/black melanin is more prevalent amongst Mediterranean and South American peoples. However, intermarriage and migration are gradually changing this picture.

There is also an association between hair colour and texture.

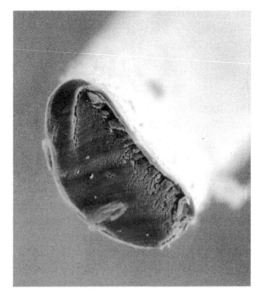

Caucasian hair cross-section

Blondes have the finest texture, whereas darker shades tend to be coarser, and redheads often have the coarsest hair. Another association is seen between hair colour and susceptibility to male hair loss. Blond males are most prone to baldness, followed by redheads and then darker shades, but the reason for this remains an evolutionary and genetic mystery. However, as a race, Caucasians are the most susceptible to male pattern hair loss.

Colour and Grooming

The diversity of colour found in Caucasian hair makes colour changes more difficult to detect. This is the group that colours its hair most frequently, and, because it greys earlier, starts colouring at a younger age.

Caucasian and Black hair are fine textured (thin in diameter), but the curl in Black hair adds body that Caucasian hair lacks. Perming and processing are the most common ways to add body. However, perming has become less popular and is now most prevalent amongst older women. They may remember it from their early days, and would need it more due to age-induced thinning or lack of effort in hair thinning management. Curly or wavy hair always has more body than straighter hair, and some waving solutions swell up the hair shaft, giving the illusion that the hair is thicker than it actually is. Likewise, all colour processes will either swell or coat the hair, or roughen the cuticle, adding further to its apparent thickness.

Caucasians love grooming products of all types but mostly use those that give body, fullness, control and thickness to their hair. Mousses, gels, sprays and lotions, either used on their own or combined, are all popular in both men and women.

Care

As a result of the above factors, Caucasian hair has more done to it, more often, than that of any other ethnic group. Special treatment is therefore important; however, the key factor is to retain the hair's body at the same time as conditioning it. This is difficult as, within the world of hair care, 'conditioner' and 'body' are sometimes considered contradictory terms, and choosing the right product in order to achieve both qualities needs careful consideration.

Unfortunately, the confusing way in which products are labelled does not make the task any easier. Ignore the terms 'oily', 'dry' and 'normal'. Instead, look for descriptions such as 'body-building', 'adding body' or 'volumizing', or, indeed, anything that suggests the way you would like your hair to be.

However, not all Caucasians have fine hair. There are those with wavier, medium-textured, coarse, curly or frizzy hair. Here again, appropriately labeled products should be chosen. Very curly or frizzy Caucasian hair needs extra moisturizing, softening, controlling and super-conditioning ingredients (see Chapter 29 on 'Formulations and Ingredients'), and a good pre-shampoo conditioner should be used as often as necessary.

For all other Caucasian hair, the following pre-shampoo conditioner can be made at home if you can't find a suitable product in the shops. Whisk in a blender:

2 eggs
2oz plain yoghurt
½oz castor oil
1oz witch hazel
1oz purified water
½ ripe avocado

Refrigerate overnight and use as necessary. Apply to the hair in sections, paying particular attention to the ends. Work the conditioner into the hair with the fingertips and then massage the scalp for a few minutes. Leave on for twenty minutes or overnight. Afterwards, shampoo and condition with your regular products. If you need to give yourself a scalp treatment, apply the scalp cream first, followed by the hair conditioner, and then massage the two together. Scalp treatments are also discussed in Chapters 8 and 22 on 'Hair Loss' and Chapter 10 on 'Dandruff'.

ORIENTAL AND ASIAN HAIR

A third distinct hair type is found in people from the continent of Asia. Although there may be minor differences between, for example, Indian, Japanese and Chinese hair, Asians can be considered as one group for hair-care purposes. An individual Asian hair has an almost perfect round shape (see photograph below) with a straight

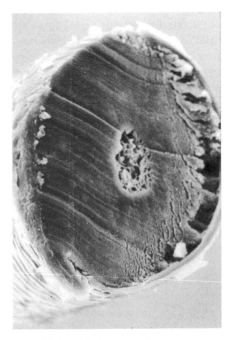

Asian/Oriental hair cross-section

or slightly wavy hair shaft. It is usually dark brown or black, has the thickest diameter of any of the ethnic groups and, moreover, is one of the strongest types of hair, with a capacity to grow to a greater length than that of other races – often over 40 inches. I have known Oriental women with hair well below the waist and even down to their ankles! The average growth rate of hair is half an inch a month, and the growth phase averages three and a half to four years, giving a length of 21–24 inches. The Oriental or Asian hair growth cycle is the longest of any group, as much as nine years, almost twice the lifespan of other hair groups. This means that the daily shedding rate is less (or should be) than that of other races, and may also account in part for the comparative infrequency of male pattern baldness amongst Oriental/Asian men, who do not suffer to the same extent as Caucasians or Blacks.

So it seems that this ethnic group has everything going for it as far as hair is concerned. Well, the males certainly have – I'm not so sure about the females. In my clinics and on visits to south-east Asia I have noticed a distinct tendency towards a general, all-over type of thinning in Oriental women, particularly over the age of forty-five. It is often unlike the recession at the front hairline, which is more common in Caucasian women. But there are not necessarily more Asian women with thinning hair, only a more pronounced thinning, which is also more noticeable because dark hair draws attention to the white scalp.

However, more research is needed to fully understand why this is and whether it is a recent phenomenon occurring only in the past twenty-five to thirty years. In that time Asian eating and living habits have become more westernized, and this may perhaps account for the different appearance and patterns found in the hair of this ethnic group. My feeling is that the change is associated with nutrition, iron and hormone levels, and also with genetic and other biological factors. Amongst some sects there is also vegetarianism, often causing low iron, low protein and other low nutrition levels. It is an interesting point that more Chinese women seem to have wavier hair in the past seven to ten years, due perhaps to eating more chicken, meat and fish, less pork and rice, but more bread.

Middle Eastern hair

This group, as previously mentioned, includes Arabic, Jewish and other Semitic races. Depending on their genetic background, it seems the incidence of a diffuse (all over) thinning, particularly affecting the top of the head, is more common than in the other ethnic groups.

Colouring and Grooming

It somehow seems unfair that Oriental/Asian hair with its thicker diameter and inherent strength to withstand the various body building and chemical processes that other ethnic types require needs them least of all. Its thickness and strength give it the natural body that Black and Caucasian hair lacks. Except, of course, when they are used to help camouflage thinning or for fashion purposes.

Greying, too, starts later in this group, making colouring (another potential weakening process) less necessary. When Oriental hair is coloured, it is usually to shades of brown or red – rarely blond, another reason why it is likely to be less abused. However, recently it seems that more Oriental women are colouring their hair blonde. Dark, straight hair reflects light, and has a shininess that curly or wavier hair often lacks. It does have a tendency towards dryness, although often this is not immediately noticeable. However, because of its larger diameter and longer length, Oriental hair is more susceptible to moisture evaporation towards the ends because they have been exposed to the elements for longer, which often leads to split and broken ends. Furthermore, long hair tends to be brushed more frequently, and while this removes dust and debris, it can also weaken the hair by removing some of the hair cuticle, making it even more vulnerable to moisture loss.

Care

It is important to minimize this loss of moisture, as Oriental/Asian hair can look quite stunning when in good condition. The use of moisturizing products and treatments is therefore essential, especially if the hair is long. Look out for the terms 'moisturizing', 'remoisturizing', 'deep conditioning' and 'elasticizing' when choosing shampoos and conditioning products. If you can't find 'extra-moisturizing' or similar on the label, then opt for products 'for dry hair'. Not the best description, I know, because 'for dry hair' can mean many things (see Chapter 4 on 'Getting to Know Your Hair'); however, such products will have moisturizing ingredients in them. And if you read Chapter 29 on 'Formulations and Ingredients' (p.156), you will have a better idea of what to look for.

Daily washing is also important. Oriental and similar hair types look wonderful when clean but can become heavy on the scalp when dirty. Do not over-dry hair with a blow dryer, or brush too hard or too often, and try to take out the tangles with a wide-toothed comb, not a brush. A weekly pre-shampoo moisturizing treatment will work wonders, and there is a wide choice of products on the market. However, if you fancy making your own, it's quite simple. Mix in blender or whisk in a bowl:

2 eggs
1oz castor oil
½oz olive oil
1oz unsalted butter
2oz double cream
1 banana (sliced thin)
Juice of a whole lemon

Refrigerate overnight if necessary. Apply the mixture to the whole length of the hair by parting in sections and then combing through with a *wide* comb. Apply extra mixture to the ends, press in with the fingers and rub lightly with the thumb and index fingers. Knead the scalp for ten minutes and press the cream into the ends again. Leave for a further ten minutes, or overnight by covering with a plastic cap. Shampoo and condition as normal, using moisturizing products.

If the scalp is flaky or itchy, or there is a hair-loss problem, apply the appropriate scalp cream first, followed by the above. Massage together as before. For more advice on scalp treatments, see Chapters 8 and 22 on 'Hair Loss' and Chapter 10 on 'Dandruff'.

For styling, control or grooming, the heavier hair-care products are rarely necessary. Light gels, mousses, protective moisturizers and leave-in conditioners are best. The inherent thickness of Oriental hair makes it easy to control, so choose a light hair spray if you wish to use one.

4

Getting to Know Your Hair

Now that I have covered many of the psychological, physiological and ethnic hair aspects, you will want to know how to deal with your own hair.

Very few people understand their hair: they are puzzled why one day their hair looks and feels good, making them happy, yet the next day they are furious because, inexplicably it seems, their hair is quite the reverse.

Many years ago I described these days by coining the phrases 'Good Hair Day' and 'Bad Hair Day'. Unfortunately, more Bad Hair Days occur than Good ones. But 'why?' you may ask. The simple answer is to understand your hair. However, it's a little more difficult than that. One of the reasons is product labels and descriptions. Although this is gradually changing, many hair products are still confusing. Everyone knows when they have dry hair, so they shop around for a shampoo or conditioner which says 'For Dry Hair'. But it's more complicated than that. Dry hair can mean many things: it can be fine, straight, limp – and dry. Or it can be coarse and curly – and dry. Or it can be very frizzy – and dry. It can even be oily at the roots – and dry at the ends. Each of these hair types could also be coloured, bleached, permed, short or long. All different but all 'Dry'.

More confusing is the term 'For Normal Hair'. What, I wonder, is 'Normal'? My 'normal', for example, would be different to your 'normal', or your relatives', friends' or children's 'normal'. Normal hair, therefore, is impossible to define. Then you may read 'For Normal/Dry Hair', 'Normal/Oily Hair', 'Normal/Coloured Hair'. These terms are even more confusing – and seemingly contradictory.

As an aside, on 'Oily' hair these days, with frequent washing an accepted requirement (rightly so), hair doesn't (or shouldn't) have the chance to get oily. Everyone produces sebum – a natural oil secreted by the sebaceous glands attached to the hair follicle – so it is 'normal' (!) for hair roots to get a little oily.

Of course, you may be lucky and choose the right combination of products for your hair, but most of you won't and will therefore be forever experimenting, becoming more confused and frustrated, with more 'Bad Hair Days' to upset you.

The only way to correctly choose is to *know* your hair and be able to describe it, look at labels and be able to think, 'Ah, yes, that's for me!'

Over twenty years ago, when I first started selling some of the products I make in my clinics, in Saks Fifth Avenue, New York, we sold out on the first day because the descriptions on the packaging – for the first time ever – said what hair type they were for. This was already easy for clients coming to my clinics, because we knew what their hair needed. It was the first time, though, that it had been done in an over-the-counter environment. Hair diameters can vary immensely, as you can see from the photograph below – some hairs being twice the thickness of others. Fine hair can be 40–70 microns in diameter (a micron is 1/1000th of a millimetre), while coarse hair can be 140 microns.

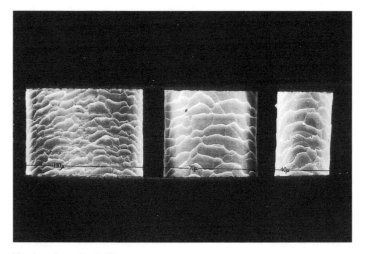

Varying sizes of hair diameter

The description on the packaging and literature accompanying them were quite simple. Since then, more accurate hair product descriptions, stating what they are for and what they are expected to do, are becoming more common. All fine or straight or limp hair, for example, needs 'body building' or 'volumizing'. Products now have these words on them or similar. Many say they are for fine hair, too. Products for curly or frizzy hair are labelled as such and would read 'remoisturizing' or 'moisturizing'. Wavy, medium textured hair about 6 inches long that has not been processed in any way may just come into the category of 'normal'. But this is so unusual now, with so many colouring agents available as well as hair being affected environmentally with sun and wind. There are products, though, for medium wavy, coloured hair, which is stated on the packaging. More usually they are 'moisture balancing'. Look at your hair carefully, think what you want it to do, read the labels and ingredients (look up Chapter 29 on 'Formulations and Ingredients' if you wish) and what they and the products claim to do – and try them. The chances are that you will be pleased. If not, try again. But you won't go far wrong if you do this.

5

Everyday Care and Maintenance

Maintaining a good-looking head of hair requires care – and care means time, a commodity that becomes increasingly more difficult. Because of this, many hair care procedures are rushed and done incorrectly. Numerous hair problems and scalp disorders can be avoided by good basic hair handling; the purpose of this chapter is to explain exactly how this should be done in the simplest and quickest possible way.

THE IMPORTANCE OF FREQUENT SHAMPOOING

The question I am asked most when a beauty editor wants to write on quick tips for hair is: 'What is the one thing that you consider most important for healthy looking hair?' Invariably, I answer, 'Daily shampooing.'

I didn't always think this. When I started in practice, in 1960, the idea of frequent shampooing didn't really occur to me. In those days, weekly washing was the norm. It was a gradual process that convinced me. I have always formulated and made my own products – shampoos included. I also introduced the concept of scalp cleansing tonics. Using a scalp tonic, for whatever purpose, resulted in the hair also getting wet. Furthermore, it meant that the active ingredients (powders and crystals) in the tonics, which were predominantly distilled water based, remained on the hair. For some types of hair this wasn't necessarily bad: for example, it gave fine, limp hair more body. However, after two to three days the hair became heavy and dirty and dull.

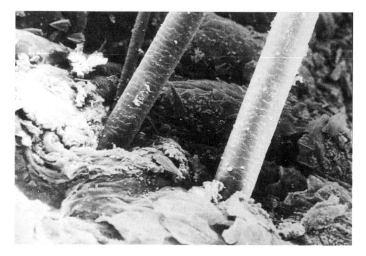

Hair and scalp 48 hours after shampooing – showing how dirty it can become

That was the beginning – I recommended washing more often to remove this unattractive 'build-up'. Not only did the hair look better (it always does when freshly shampooed), but the effect of the scalp tonic was enhanced and the overall improvement on whatever the problem became more apparent.

It didn't take long to convince me that the more the hair is shampooed, the better it responded, as well as giving the hair a superior image and improved styling and control capabilities. Using a beneficial scalp tonic wet the hair and spoiled its style anyway, so it was no big deal going a stage further and *really* wetting the hair with shampooing! It also occurred to me that everybody washes their face once a day, so why not the hair? You take your hair to the same places and it gets just as dirty!

Shampooing: The Art and Skill

If you follow these steps, you will find you will begin to benefit immediately. Don't rush – the difference between correct and incorrect is less than a minute.

Dry Run

Run a wide-toothed comb through the hair before wetting, as it follows that if you start with tangles, you'll end up with more tangles.

Remove tangles from the ends first, then gradually work up the hair shafts.

Pre-Soaking

This is vital. Thoroughly wet hair will need less shampoo. Use warm water and gently draw your fingers through your hair as the water is flowing over it.

Applying Shampoo and Lathering

A potentially good technique can often go wrong here. Instead of pouring the shampoo directly onto the hair, pour it onto the palm of your hand, rub your hands together and then smooth the shampoo over your hair. Gently rub your palms over your hair, then massage the scalp with the fingertips in a gentle kneading motion. Be careful to avoid scratching your scalp with your fingernails, and do not use a massage brush. Continue the massaging action for approximately thirty seconds and every so often run your fingers through your hair from front to back in order to avoid tangling.

Rinse

This should be done for longer than you think is necessary. Even when you think you have rinsed sufficiently, rinse again. A common cause of dull hair is insufficient rinsing, and contrary to popular belief, there is no reason to finish off a rinse with cold water unless you enjoy it. One lathering is all that is necessary when washing your hair daily. Otherwise, give two latherings by repeating the above procedure.

CONDITIONING, OVER-CONDITIONING AND THEIR EFFECT ON HAIR 'BODY'

Considering there is no such thing as over-conditioning, it is extraordinary how often this mythical hazard is mentioned. To have hair that is 'over-conditioned' is like being 'overhealthy'.

To condition hair literally means to improve its condition. Shampooing cleanses but at the same time often tangles hair, because it can cause the cuticles (the outer cells of the hair) to interlock with the cells of another hair. A conditioner will smooth these cells and therefore help to avoid tangles, also giving extra shine. Confusion can arise when those with limp or thin, fine hair find that it loses body after conditioning. This is likely to be the result either of using the wrong conditioner for your hair type or of incorrect use and too little rinsing. On the other hand, with thick, curly hair, over-conditioning is unheard of.

It is always advisable to use an after-shampoo conditioner whatever your hair type. Pour a small quantity into the palm of your hand, rub your hands together and smooth the conditioner over the hair, paying particular attention to the ends. Do not rub into the scalp or put the conditioner on the hair near the scalp. Rinse immediately. There is no reason to leave conditioner in your hair for any length of time. A well-formulated conditioner should act on the hair instantly. After thoroughly rinsing, rinse again. Conditioners used after shampooing are primarily formulated for de-tangling and smoothing, and leaving them in too long is pointless. There are conditioning products that are intended to be left in, but I will discuss these in other sections.

When you have finished, wrap the hair in a towel and press this against your head with your hands to absorb surplus moisture. Follow by gently removing tangles with a wide-toothed comb, starting at the ends.

Hair 'Body'

In order to avoid loss of body, it is important that the right conditioner is used in the right way. Your choice of product is the key to successful conditioning. In Chapter 3 on 'The Ethnic Behaviour of Hair' and Chapter 4 on 'Getting to Know Your Hair' I have made recommendations for the various hair types. Those of you whose hair needs extra body should choose your product carefully. If you have fine, limp hair that has been over-processed, you will have to choose between counteracting the damage with a high-moisturizing product, which while increasing the hair's softness may reduce body, or using a body-building conditioner, which while adding body will not be of sufficient help in de-tangling or in moisturizing.

The best alternative is to use a high-moisturizing product and then a conditioning styling aid that adds volume and body. There are a good variety of such products on the market. Styling aids also have the advantage of being able to vary the quantity used according to how much body you require. I hasten to add that this is not over-conditioning but sensible conditioning (see also Chapter 14 on 'Styling Your Hair Safely').

6

Brushes and Combs

Generally speaking, it is better to use a comb rather than a brush, as it's a lot harder to comb your hair vigorously and therefore your movements tend to be gentler. If you use a brush, be careful when choosing it. A woman who came to me complaining of hair loss and a sore scalp proudly showed me her brush. It was beautifully made with polished wood and pure bristles. The bristles had tiny metal prongs in the center of each tuft and it really did look wonderful. She said that she had been using it to stimulate her scalp and remove her dandruff. Unfortunately, the brush did neither: it was full of hair and her scalp was full of scratches.

Vigorous brushing, whatever is used, weakens the hair by removing some of the hair's cuticle – the outer cell layer. It breaks it off and, by constant traction, pulls the hair out. Furthermore, sharp points remove the top layer of skin. An exaggeration? Not at all. The damage a brush can cause is severely underrated.

I am not trying to scare you off using a brush – it is often an essential styling tool – but you need to be careful.

Choose a brush with long, widely spaced, plastic (not natural) bristle, as plastic bristles are smoother, blunter and kinder. Natural bristles are sharper, often barbed and are tufted close together. Above all, avoid anything with metal prongs. Apart from being kinder to your hair, plastic brushes are kinder to your pocket. The difference in price can be incredible.

Brushing hair should never be regarded as a means of exercising it. Try brushing your wool sweater or dress fifty times a day and see how quickly it wears out! Also, do not pull at tangles after shampooing: it is better to remove them with a comb, starting at the ends. Wet hair becomes swollen and stretched (often by as much as 20–30 per cent). Over-zealous brushing can therefore snap the hair like a rubber band. To avoid this, use your brush gently and do not pull or twist your hair too much when blow drying.

Although combing may not always give you as much control over your style, a comb is easier on the hair, provided you are using the right type. You may wonder what the difference is between one comb and another. Just as with brushes, there are good ones and bad ones. Many combs, particularly the cheaper, plastic types, are made in a mould and have join lines down the inner center of each tooth where the mould comes together. These lines can cut the hair shaft, remove cells and, eventually, weaken the hair. Metal combs are even worse, as their edges can lacerate the hair.

I would recommend that you use a 'saw-cut' comb, in which each tooth is cut into the comb, making them smoother. The standard substance from which saw-cut combs are made is vulcanite (a type of hard rubber), but some good plastic saw-cut combs are also available. Vulcanite is better because of its anti-static properties and because they are easier to clean. A disadvantage is their colour – usually black, like a hairdresser's comb, and they don't look attractive on the dressing table or in the bathroom. If you look hard enough, though, you may find them in other colours.

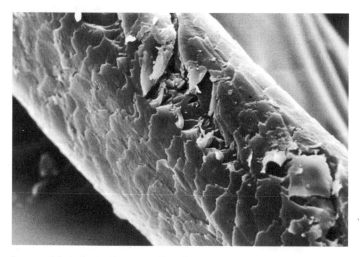

Lacerated hair from using a metal comb

The best styling results are obtained when using a comb to ease out tangles and a brush to style the hair into shape whilst using the blow dryer.

It is vital when using brushes and combs to make sure they are cleaned regularly, as they are prone to collect dirt. One of the best ways to do this is to dissolve a tablespoon of washing soda in a basin of water, add a little antiseptic and then tap the brush or comb briskly in it. You'll be surprised at how much dirt comes out. Afterwards, rinse with clean water.

7

The Rules of Hair Growth

To enable a better understanding of hair thinning and hair loss, which comes up again and again in discussing Chapters 8 and 22 on 'Hair Loss', I have coined another phrase: 'The Rules of Hair Growth'. It's not going to become the classic 'Bad Hair Day' I started over twenty-five years ago, but it's a phrase which sums up the misunderstanding connected with what occurs during the time between seemingly having a full head of hair and then a noticeably thinner one.

It is impossible to calculate the number of occasions when a woman or man has sat in my consulting room complaining of thinning hair, convinced that it started only six months or so ago.

Except in cases of post-partum hair fall or hair fall as a consequence of a high fever, illness or chemotherapy, whereby the hair is rapidly and frighteningly shed in huge amounts, it is impossible for hair to thin noticeably in just six months – particularly when the hair's shedding rate doesn't seem to have changed that much.

There may be the possibility that the shedding rate *has* increased, but more often than not it's when the thinning is first noticed that the amount of hair coming out is looked at more closely. And a normal amount of fall becomes worrisome and is viewed as being excessive.

Alternatively, many people may say that they can't understand why their hair has thinned, as it doesn't seem to be coming out much!

The unfortunate fact of hair thinning is that you need to lose about 15 per cent of hair volume before it is even noticed – and unless it has been coming out in really huge quantities as mentioned, it is impossible for hair to thin 15 per cent in six months.

Sometimes, for no apparent reason, there may be a temporary

increase in the hair's shedding rate. It could be seasonal – or it could be inexplicable. It may last a month or six weeks or more, then just as inexplicably stop. This also brings extra attention to whatever hair thinning has taken place previously.

A 'Hair Growth Rule' is that hair remains in its growth phase for approximately four years. It fluctuates with race and individuals. At the end of its growth phase, the hair is shed; three months later another grows in its place. For anybody to notice a difference in their hair volume (15 per cent less) without a lot of hair fall, it must have began three to four years earlier – not just the six months of complaining.

Another rule: if the hair has considerably reduced in volume, another few years could be added in. Assume (as an analogy) that each hair starts the diameter of a 'thumb' and grows for four years at 6 inches a year. If left uncut, it would grow 24 inches, fall out and three months later be replaced by another hair that may be only a 'finger' diameter and grow for just two and a half to three years. This in turn may be replaced by a 'little finger' hair (pinkie) growing for two years. We already have a minimum of eight years of thinning (or reduced volume). But very thinned hair could take even longer, the hairs becoming thinner and thinner in diameter and eventually growing shorter and shorter in length, many reaching the 'non-meaningful' stage when the hairs are so fine and short that you can't see them. They don't mean anything to the overall appearance. This can take ten or twenty years.

A woman's noticeable thinning at the front and generally over the scalp or a man's receding hair line and thinning on the crown

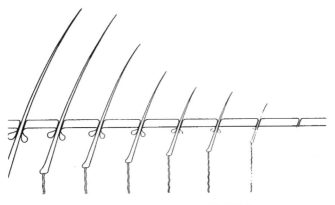

CHANGES IN GROWTH OVER TIME

could not possibly have taken only six months – six years may be more accurate depending on genetic factors and the rate of hair shedding.

The point I am making is that thinning hair starts long before you become aware of it. It could (and often does) start in the early teens – gradually and almost remorselessly. I mention in another chapter that the hairs' peak of volume is just before or after puberty.

I do not mean to alarm you by saying all this – you may not be in this category. However, gradual change is one of the rules of hair growth, particularly if you are genetically prone.

Although I will refer further to this throughout the book, it does make another important point: it's never too early to start taking care.

8

Hair Loss in Women

There is so much to say on this subject that it is difficult to know exactly where to begin – and what age to begin with (see previous chapter).

It can begin at puberty, when pregnant, after childbirth, menopause, with taking oral contraceptives or HRT. The common denominator in all these is a change in hormones – oestrogens and androgens. But there is much more than just the involvement of hormones, as you will see later.

Those of you with thinning hair know only too well how much distress it causes, and not a day goes by in my practice without a distraught woman in despair because of her thinning hair.

Not long ago, a popular newspaper reported on 'The plague of hair loss' amongst women, arguing that because women have taken a more aggressive (and male) role, they must therefore suffer with male health disorders, of which hair loss is one.

But is there more female hair loss now than ever before? It is impossible to gauge whether there has been an increase. There is no doubt that more women are complaining of hair loss, but this doesn't mean that there *is* more. Certainly there has been a progressive increase in press coverage, making women more aware and thus encouraging more of them to seek advice. The plethora of so-called 'hair growing miracles' adds to this awareness. With my practice, and that of colleagues, the incidence of women seeking advice has certainly increased, but we can't compare it to ten or twenty or thirty years ago because there are no true statistics.

I have commented for many years that the incidence of hair loss in females is seriously underestimated and that hair thinning in women is as common as it is in men but without the extreme form of baldness. Indeed, although I have seen a few women with hair loss bordering on male baldness, it is rare.

There was a time, and it still exists to a great extent, when a woman wouldn't mention hair thinning. It was, and still remains (perhaps less so), a taboo subject, with connotations of being unfeminine, unattractive, ageing and masculine. Gradually, it seems that women are thinking about it differently. And rightly so.

I would need to have my arm twisted quite hard to give my opinion on the purported extra occurrence of women's hair loss. Assuming it has been twisted hard, I may give a 'probably' but not a definitely. It may well be connected to the extra stresses women are experiencing, which can cause hair loss, but also to the various hormone medications: oral contraceptives and hormone replacement therapies (HRT). But more about those later.

Hormones play a huge part and there has been one outstanding addition to our knowledge recently: PCOS.

PCOS (POLYCYSTIC OVARIAN SYNDROME)

I started my clinic in New York in 1977. Two or three years later, when I seemed to be successful, a woman was recommended to me by her doctor husband because of her thinning hair. After seeing her, I referred her back to her husband for specific blood tests to verify my suspicions. Consequently, I eventually met the doctor and began a relationship I consider to be one of the most important in my professional career – as well as making a true friend. His name is Dr Walter Futterweit, a Clinical Professor of Endocrinology.

We began cross-referring patients, and over time a pattern started to emerge in young women of reproductive age – women still having periods – all of them complaining of thinning or falling hair (or both, because they are not necessarily the same). We eventually became involved in a clinical study with two others: Dr Andrea Dunaif and Dr Hsu-Chong Yeh. In essence, of 109 women with an average age of thirty-two, about 30 per cent had PCOS – and the prevailing, if not the only, symptom was hair loss, which was the only reason the women had sought advice. At the time it was estimated that about 10 per cent of women suffered from PCOS. The original name was Polycystic Ovarian Disease (PCOD), but it's not a disease

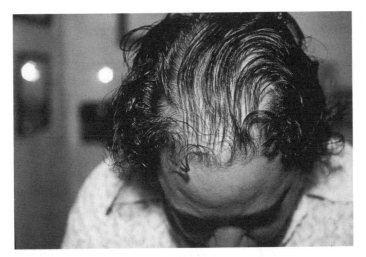

An example of hair loss resulting from Polycystic Ovarian Syndrome

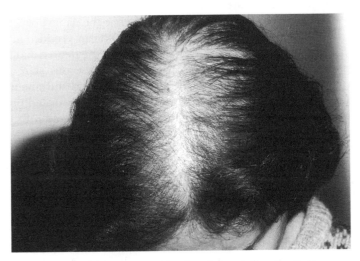

Another example of hair loss resulting from Polycystic Ovarian Syndrome

as much as a syndrome, a combination of symptoms, with hair loss being one of them. Other symptoms include irregular menstrual cycles, difficulty in conceiving, extra hair on the face and body, acne, greasy skin, being overweight and having diabetes mellitus.

Since then, I and several other doctors have just completed another study that is almost ready for publication. However, the results are even more surprising than the first study. Of 89 women of similar ages to the first study, 67 per cent had PCOS – an enormously high percentage.

Although all women in both studies sought advice for thinning hair as the only symptom, the original estimate of 10–12 per cent of women suffering from PCOS is almost certainly underestimated (as, indeed, is the percentage of women suffering from hair loss). (See photographs p.35.)

PCOS is not dangerous or life-threatening, although the anxiety it causes can result in serious depression and ruin a person's quality of life. And the name, polycystic ovaries, sounds worse than it really is. All ovaries have small undulations over their surface like small peaks and valleys, and these are called follicles. When the follicles become more pronounced they appear cyst-like – hence the name polycystic ovaries. It is actually an endocrine disorder and can produce more androgens (male hormones). Androgens affect the degree and frequency of bleeding in the menstrual cycle, cause oily skin and tendency to acne, grow hair where you don't want it and diminish growth where you do. However, as with so many hair-related problems, it's not that simple. Genetic susceptibility enters into the equation. Extra androgens have a greater detrimental effect on those with hair follicles that are more sensitive to their presence. For example, a woman with little or no hair follicle sensitivity could be affected very little by extra androgens, whereas one with high sensitivity could be affected by normal or even subnormal amounts.

Yet PCOS hair loss is predominately dependent on more androgens being produced – the term used being hyperandrogenism.

Treatment for PCOS can be complicated, depending on symptoms other than thinning hair. But if hair loss is the only or predominant symptom, it is relatively straightforward, treated by the ingestion of anti-androgens. The most common one used is Spironolactone (Aldactone) or Dianette, an oral contraceptive. Recent research indicates that women with PCOS may be more prone to heart disease and have a greater tendency to diabetes mellitis. Reduction of dietary fat and carbohydrates can improve symptoms. Metformin, a drug that decreases the body's requirement for insulin, can also be effective. However, drugs taken orally are often insufficiently effective on the 'target site', in this case the hair follicle, and topical (externally applied) solutions are needed on the scalp itself. Containing anti-androgens, they can be extremely effective.

None of the treatments mentioned can be obtained over-the-counter. They need a qualified person to dispense them. It is also important to bear in mind that even if PCOS is a culprit in hair thinning, it may only be one of them. Do not overlook other aspects that may be causative, all of which you will read about later on.

THE PILL (ORAL CONTRACEPTIVE)

One of the medications for PCOS is Dianette – an oral contraceptive. It's an anti-androgen and contains the potent anti-androgen, *cyproterone acetate*. It is not available in the USA yet, but easily obtained in the UK, Europe and Canada (Dianne). For some types of hair shedding and thinning, it can be helpful – and so can many other oral contraceptives. However, others could be detrimental.

The Pill is no doubt the easiest and most reliable form of contraception. Most contain two hormones: oestrogen and progestin (some only a progestin). They inhibit ovulation, each of the two hormones able to do this job by themselves, although a combination is usually preferred.

As far as hair is concerned, there are many myths connected to oral contraceptives: I see many women aged twenty to forty who blame the Pill for their hair fall or hair thinning because it had been noticeable only since they started taking it. This type of self-diagnosis is very common, as it makes a person feel better if they can put the blame on something, stop what they think is the cause and all will be well again. Many women had done this: they had stopped taking the Pill and started again when they saw it made no difference or, indeed, led to increased hair fall (coming off the Pill can result in a type of post-partum shedding).

Some writers have blamed the Pill for the apparent increase in female hair loss. After all, the thinking goes that the Pill has been in existence for over forty years, so it must be one of the culprits!

To my knowledge there has been no published medical or scientific studies comparing pre-Pill to post-Pill days. There is an argument, though, for the assumption that the Pill increases the tendency to thinner hair. Some may do so but others would not and can even have a beneficial rather than detrimental effect.

A complication of comparison is the range of susceptibility of each person's hair follicles, too. Some women have greater hair follicle sensitivity than others – and this is usually genetic.

There are some guidelines to consider if you are thinking of starting on the Pill, coming off it or changing to another brand of the type you are already on if you feel (or see) a potential hair thinning problem.

The past few years has seen an increase in 'less androgenic' combinations. A Pill with more androgens would be less desirable than one with a smaller percentage or a compound that in itself has a more androgenic effect.

The following is a guide that may influence your choice. Ones that may be considered more androgenic include those that contain Norethisterone, Levonorgestrel, Gestodene and Ethynodiol Diacetate. The better ones include those containing Medroxyprogesterone Acetate, Desorgestrol, Norgestimate, Ethinyloestradiol and Cyproterone Acetate (the last being unavailable in the USA, but available in Canada and most other countries). The Pills have different brand names but the active ingredients are on the package, so look at them carefully.

It goes without saying that you need to discuss your choice with your doctor or gynaecologist, and as these are guidelines, it is possible that the Pill best for your hair may not be suitable for your metabolism.

PREGNANCY

The misunderstandings and general mythology on the effects of pregnancy on your hair are countless.

Your hair is always important, but it will become even more so as soon as you know that you're pregnant. It will take on a new meaning and, more than ever, you will want it to look wonderful and to use it as a sexual characteristic to enhance your appearance, particularly towards the end of your pregnancy.

A few years ago I helped in a study entitled 'The effect of pregnancy on scalp hair and facial skin'. We studied 375 women for three years. It won't come as a surprise to you to learn that the most frequently asked question was, 'How will pregnancy affect my hair?'

The popular press has endorsed the theory that pregnancy is a terrific time for hair; it sometimes is and sometimes isn't. Although skin changes are often noticeable within weeks of conception, changes in the hair are not. As hair has a growth rate of half an inch a month, it wouldn't be possible to notice changes so rapidly (except that there may be changes in the amount of sebum produced by your sebaceous glands, and this can effect the hair's appearance and feel).

We discovered that approximately 50 per cent of women had post-partum fall.

About a third of the pregnant women questioned in the study did see an improvement in their hair after four to five months, saying it fell out less and felt thicker. This lasted for the rest of the pregnancy. Hormonal changes during pregnancy, which include an increase in oestrogen levels and a diminishing of androgens, can cause a decrease in the production of sebum. An over-oily scalp can give the hair a heavy, limp and lanky feel, and it is the acidity of sebum that smoothes down the hair's cuticle. When less sebum is produced, the hair appears to be drier and to have more body, so it feels thicker. Although the hair may look better, its condition has not really improved. However, oestrogens do extend the growth phase of hair, so it stays in the scalp and grows longer. This is certainly not an illusion.

On the other hand, a third of the women questioned stated the opposite! The remaining third did not notice any difference.

We also tried to connect poor hair conditions and post-partum fall with the incidence of morning sickness, but there was no correlation at all. So why some women have wonderful hair during pregnancy and others complain of it all the time is still puzzling. We know that hormonal changes during pregnancy vary and that the susceptibility of the hair follicles to these changes also varies. It is impossible to estimate in advance what the effects will be. We know that if your hair is wonderful during your first pregnancy, it could be quite the reverse during the second – or vice versa. What is certain is that women with two, three or more children tend to have less hair than women with one child. But don't let that put you off! A woman with only one child is usually younger, so the age factor should be taken into account.

Many women also notice that their hair is terrible for the first three to four months of their pregnancy and then a miraculous change appears to occur. To make you feel better, and also because it's true, I must say that it is rare for a woman to have problems with her hair all through the nine months. The last three months in particular should be very good for your hair.

So what can you do to ensure you get the best from your hair during these nine months? Firstly, without being told, you will automatically begin to take more care of yourself. You will eat better, do what your doctor tells you and take the supplements he gives you. You should also be less stressed, knowing you shouldn't overexert yourself.

A growing foetus uses a huge amount of energy and, consequently, you will get tired more often, so you will need to rest whenever possible. You must follow the four-hour nutrition rule, i.e. snack on a piece of fruit if you leave more than four hours between meals. Your hair is not essential tissue like your growing baby, so it will suffer is you don't eat regularly.

As previously mentioned, it is likely that your hair will feel progressively drier during your pregnancy. Give it an occasional drink with a moisturizing, pre-shampoo deep-conditioner. You may also need to change your shampoo or conditioner temporarily to one with a deeper moisturizing factor. Wash your hair every day, as it will look its best if clean. Go easy on the brush and don't over-dry it with the hair dryer. Use whatever styling aids make you happy and have whatever style you want – pregnancy is rather a good time to experiment. You can perm, straighten, colour or bleach your hair if you wish.

Above all, don't worry about your hair. Apart from a hiccup or two at the beginning, by the end of your pregnancy, the chances are that your hair will look great!

MENOPAUSE

Continuing the subject of hair loss in women, there is a need to focus further on the hormonal aspect. The last two sections on PCOS and pregnancy are really examples of what hormone changes can do to hair growth. PCOS is a condition associated with younger women, since it can begin at puberty. Pregnancy is usually later and can continue into the mid-forties. But hormone changes causing the most distress are those that occur with menopause. The changes also almost always affect the hair.

The average age of menopause is around fifty but symptoms can begin long before. Apart from the more associated common symptoms of 'hot flushes' and discomfort, the skin begins to appear a little drier and not as elastic. This is quite easily countered by applying moisturizers, and I am sure that moisturizing cosmetics are used progressively more pre- and post-menopausally. The changes in the hair, though, are more difficult to counteract. They may begin with a heavier shedding rate or a noticed reduction in thickness (volume). Not straight away – it's gradual. Reduction in hair volume, however, often begins long before menopause, with menopause being an extra and more accelerating cause. Not only that, from a psychological viewpoint more women begin to look even closer at themselves – they think they are now *really* ageing – and want to find more fault to prove their fears. The psychology of being unable to bear another child is an important aspect. However, a woman's role does not diminish with menopause. At fifty she is still young and active and can be as attractive as she was a decade or more earlier.

Without delving further into other physiological changes, the change affecting a woman most is that which occurs with her hair. Hair is deeply psychologically sexual, and the feeling of insecurity in her sexuality with all the accompanying changes is further undermined with those in the hair.

The basis of all these changes is diminishing oestrogens.

Except for the time before puberty, oestrogens (and therefore androgens) .become a greater issue throughout a woman's life. They effect frequency of the menstrual cycle, the type of menstruation (heavy, light, long, short), sexual arousal and appetite, mood swings, skin and, of course, hair.

The diminishing oestrogens affect the cycle of hair growth – oestrogens prolong it. As the secretion of oestrogens slows down, so does the length to which the hair will grow. Additionally, androgens increase as a percentage. Androgens can cause extra facial and body hair and lessen scalp hair – not necessarily in numbers, but in diameter and length, resulting in a loss of volume or 'body'. The hair fall could remain as it was but the replacement hairs become progressively weaker. This occurs slowly, not suddenly happen with menopause. The changes in oestrogen secretion do not occur overnight either – they are also gradual. It is inevitable that changes in hair volume begin long before the physical manifestations of menopause are noticed. But it is not unusual for women to blame the short time of, say, six months, when they first begin to realize that menopausal changes were occurring for their lack of hair.

I have for many years stated that nobody over forty has the same volume of hair they had in their twenties. So if the average age of menopause is fifty, changes would begin to occur in the early forties anyway.

The pattern of hair thinning tends to be similar to the early stages of male pattern hair loss – that is, a recession at the frontal hair line and temples. *Not* less hair in numbers, but smaller diameters and shorter growth. Sometimes a diffuse (generalized, overall) loss can occur, too. I can't even attempt to guess at the number of women I have seen who have been in a state of near hysteria because of their diminishing hair. 'I'm going to be bald like a man,' is the cry I so often hear. Of course, they're not; even with neglect, it is very rare for women to go bald. Yet the degree of anxiety the thought causes should not be underestimated.

You will no doubt be wondering how an apparently natural change such as menopause can be counteracted in your hair: it can, perhaps not wholly, but certainly considerably, an issue I will discuss later.

HORMONE REPLACEMENT THERAPY (HRT)

The dilemma of whether to have hormone replacement therapy continues. Studies have shown that there is the possibility of side effects such as breast cancer, heart problems, mood swings, greater tendency to cancer of the uterus and endometriosis. It all sounds frightening but the figures are rather misleading. The risks appear to be greater but the percentages are small. It is then a matter of choice – whether to alleviate the unpleasant symptoms that cause a lesser quality of life or to run the small extra risks associated with the side effects to enable you to lead a better and more comfortable existence. And often help your hair at the same time.

The choices of HRT can be confusing and complicated, and most women are guided by their doctor or gynaecologist, very few understanding or considering the effect of the medication on hair. Some can be detrimental whilst others can be beneficial. Another potential problem is that different women respond in different ways to the same HRT, and a few changes might be necessary before the correct combination is found, the result sometimes not being ultimately conducive to hair.

Guidelines

Basically, hormone replacement therapy is administered to restore circulating levels of oestrogen to average pre-menopausal levels in order to relieve menopausal symptoms and reduce the risk of osteoporosis.

HYSTERECTOMY

A hysterectomy is the surgical removal of the womb, which may or may not include the removal of the ovaries. In either case, oestrogens may be administered alone. When a hysterectomy has not taken place, a progestogen must be added to the oestrogen therapy for ten to fourteen days at the end of each cycle to protect the endometrium (membrane lining the womb) against the greater cell reproduction that leads to cancer.

The oestrogen only HRTs for women without a uterus (womb) are numerous, and examples include Adgyn Estro, Climaval, Dermerstril, Elleste-Solo, Estraderm, Estradiol Implants, Evorel, Fimatrix, Femseven, Menorest, Oestrogel, Premarin, Progynova, Sandrena and Zumenon.

HRT preparations with oestrogens plus a progesterone derivative *and* that can be beneficial to hair include Premique, Indivina and Tridestra. All contain medroxyprogesterone acetate – usually a goodie as far as hair is concerned. Others, such as Femapak and Femoston, contain dydrogesterone – another goodie. Sometimes Premarin is given, which is oestrogen combined with Proveral as the progestogen. The combination may also be beneficial to hair.

Progestogens

As a further guideline, these are synthetic compounds with actions similar to those of natural progesterone. Both are hormones. There are two main groups of progestogens. All possess androgenic activity (you have already read that androgens can be detrimental to hair), however progesterone (and similar hormones) have less androgens than progestogens.

The choice of HRTs with progestogens that have a greater androgen effect is also quite large. In the main – and if possible – they should be avoided due to their possible deleterious effect on the hair. These include Adgyn Combi, Climagest, Climesse, Ellest-Duet,

Estracombi, Estrapak 50, Evorel Pak, Kliofem, Kliovance and Trisequens. The progestrogen in these is Norethisterone. Another possible adverse progestogen is Levonorgestrol, which is contained in Cyclo-Progynova and Nuvelle. Livial, which contains Tibilone, a combined oestrogen and progestogen, is thought to have androgenic activity, too.

So, to sum up, the compounds to look for with regard to being hair-favourable are Dydrogesterone, Hydroxyprogesterone, Medroxyprogesterone and Natural Progesterone. Unfavourable to hair are Norgestrel, Desogestrel, Norgestinate and Gestodene. And the two *most unfavourable* are Norethisterone and Levonorgestral.

I hope this rather complicated list has been simplified sufficiently to enable you to make an easier choice. However, your doctor must be consulted, although a little knowledge of 'hair adversaries' in the choice of HRT could convince him or her in their recommendation.

Hair is not the only factor to be considered, although if you do have a hair thinning problem, you will no doubt be distressed and your doctor should be made aware of it to try to influence their choice.

9

Babies, Toddlers, Infants and Children

Hair from Birth to Puberty and Teens

In a way it might have been sensible to have this chapter at the beginning of the book, but it's not that clear cut. Perhaps after the pregnancy section in the Women's Hair Loss chapter would have been better. Again, it doesn't quite work, so here we are!

I have already mentioned the unfortunate fact that 50 per cent of women have post-partum hair loss. However, I did not discuss the effects on the other 50 per cent.

There is no doubt that one of the prime concerns in the vast majority of women after pregnancy is their hair. By focusing on their own hair, adding to the stresses of bringing up a baby, poor baby's hair is often an afterthought. 'What can go wrong with a baby's hair?' they may think. Well, not a lot in reality, but there are aspects you should bear in mind and certainly rules that should be followed.

BABIES

Firstly, a baby is born with a specific number of hair follicles, which control how much hair they will have throughout their life and whether their hair will be fine, medium, coarse, straight, wavy or curly. These factors can't be changed, as they are all genetically predetermined. Many babies are born with barely any noticeable hair whilst others have quite a crop. If your baby looks bald, don't worry: the hair will grow eventually. The time it takes varies enormously, and mothers have brought their one and two year olds to me, worried that they have so little hair. Hair, though, is as individual as walking, talking or becoming potty-trained – when the time is right, the hair will grow.

A newborn baby's scalp is not fully formed. At the top of the head (the crown) the skull bones have not yet completely knitted together, leaving a 'soft spot' – almost an indentation. Baby's scalp bones are also soft. As a consequence, mothers are often afraid to wash their baby's hair for fear of injury. However, the scalp should be bathed along with the rest of the baby.

How to Shampoo Babies' Hair

The best way is to gently ladle warm water onto the scalp with the palms of your hands and pour a little of your own shampoo diluted (one part in five with purified water) onto one palm. Rub your palms together and with the flat of your hands gently caress your baby's scalp until the shampoo lathers, then rinse it off by ladling more warm water onto it again.

You may wonder why you should use your own shampoo and not a 'baby' shampoo. The answer is that what suits you will usually suit your baby. Also, so-called 'baby' shampoos (what a wonderful name – it automatically denotes mildness) did not compare well when tested against 'adult' shampoos. I blind tested numerous shampoos, including baby shampoo, for my first book, and I'm sorry to say that baby shampoo didn't get good marks. It is true that they don't sting the eyes, but that doesn't necessarily mean they are better for the hair.

Frequency of Shampooing Babies' Hair and Cradle Cap

Similarly to your own, it should be washed daily. If your baby's hair is not washed frequently, the natural scalp secretions and skin shedding can congeal into a rather unsightly yellow-brown covering of flakes called 'cradle cap'. This can look quite unattractive, with some babies being more prone to it than others. Moreover, the latest scientific opinion suggests that some types of milk can be a factor in this condition, in which case a change in milk formula could help. Likewise, if for some reason mother's milk isn't suitable, a change to a milk formula bottle could be beneficial.

Cradle cap may develop if you neglect the daily washing of your baby's scalp or it may develop for other reasons: the baby may be unduly sensitive or, as has been suggested, parents with chronic dandruff (see Chapter 10) are more likely to have babies who are extra prone to cradle cap. Either way, cradle cap can be easily removed. Warm a little light vegetable oil and gently dab it on the scalp with a cotton wool ball. Leave on for five to ten minutes and dab the scalp similarly with diluted (one part in five) shampoo. Rub the scalp gently with the palms of the hands in a circular movement, ladle more water to get a lather and gently rub this with the palms of your hands too. Finally, rinse off by ladling more warm water from your palms to the head. The number of times you will need to do this will depend upon how much cradle flaking there is. You will need to do it every day for a few days to remove the cradle cap if it is very congealed. When clear, it is a good idea to do the process occasionally anyway. This, too, will depend on the baby's tendency to produce the condition.

TODDLERS, INFANTS AND CHILDREN TO PRE-PUBERTY

As your baby gets older, washing hair becomes more difficult. Most children hate it because either the shampoo stings the eyes or water gets into them. However, it is essential to keep the hair and scalp clean. A good way to get over an infant's dislike of hair washing is to turn it into a game. Give them a face cloth to hold over their eyes and ask them to guess where you are going to touch their head first or where most water will be felt and so on, a bit like blind man's bluff.

To avoid tangles do not rub the hair too hard and always use a conditioner. It is odd that often mothers do not consider it necessary to use a conditioner on their child's hair. On the contrary, it's just as important as it is for adults, particularly if the hair is long or has been exposed to sun, wind, pool water or beach life. Comb the hair gently and never brush it hard. Also avoid tight clips and ponytails with tightly wound bare elastic bands – all of these can lead to hair breakage and traction hair loss.

The toddler and infant stages end at about three years old, and up until this age it is advisable to use a diluted version of your own shampoo. Pour 1oz (30ml) into a bottle and add 4oz (120ml) of purified water. Shake well and use as necessary. After the age of two and until the age of five, the percentage of shampoo can be increased to 50 per cent, then 75 per cent and full strength at five or six. This is what I did with my daughters, now aged nineteen and twenty-two, and their hair is wonderful.

CHILDREN FROM 5 TO 11 (PRE-PUBERTY)

As your child grows up, his or her hair will begin to change. A baby's hair is very fine and has a small diameter – which is not surprising considering the size of the host. The hair's diameter gradually increases from birth to two years, growing rather rapidly up until the age of four or five, then begins to slow down. By the age of ten or eleven, when puberty is on the near horizon, the scalp hairs have reached their full diameter – a little earlier in girls than boys.

Up until puberty, hair is relatively trouble-free, assuming you take reasonable care. This is really quite easy: children rarely have chemical processing such as bleach (unless from sun), colour, perming, tugging when blow-drying, tight ponytails or hair pulled back too tightly. Ordinary daily shampooing and conditioning should keep it in good shape.

Nits and Lice (Pediculosis)

This is more common than realized amongst school children. It's odd that this infestation is almost always referred to as 'nits' and hardly ever as 'lice'. I suppose 'nit' sounds more genteel. But obviously you have to have a living louse to lay the eggs (which are the nits) in the first place.

Lice are greyish white in colour and sometimes brown, particularly when they have had a feed of your blood (sorry about this), and you have to peer very closely to see them, as they are only about 3mm long, with the male being slightly smaller than the female. The female lives for about a month and lays seven to ten eggs a day, which hatch in a week into 'nymphs'. The nymphs reach maturity in eight days or so. Nymphs and adults suck blood from the scalp and in doing so inject their saliva into the skin, causing itching; the scratching often removes the louse, which can then be seen under your nail.

Lice are not necessarily the result of dirt, although poor hygiene can be a factor, as this means that not enough overall care is being taken. Private schools are as prone to outbreaks as state schools, and infestation is more common in girls than boys because of their longer hair. It is also thought that girls' sweat and sebum secretions are possibly more to the louse's liking as well.

The only way to catch lice is through direct contact, either through shared combs, brushes, hats or even chair backs. The stigma attached to 'having nits' is very strong, but it is really no different than catching any other infection such as a cold. Furthermore, they are much easier to cure than a cold. A couple of applications (or even one application) of a shampoo or lotion made for this purpose usually kills them off. However, lice, which have been in existence for as long as we have, rapidly acquire a resistance to a specific medication, in which case changing to another should do the trick. Your doctor or chemist will advise you on this.

Removing the nits from the hair is bothersome. They are dead after the application of the 'nit killer', but they remain unattractively stuck on the hair shaft. A nit comb is used for this – a comb with very narrow teeth, which dislodges the nit as it is combed through the hair. It can be laborious and time-consuming.

There has been some controversy on the side effects of the drugs used in louse shampoos and lotions, most containing Malathion, with many warnings. However, shampooing the hair, following with a creamy conditioner and not rinsing it out to leave the hair slippery, then using the nit comb, can also be quite effective and has no possible side effects. This needs to be done once or twice a day for two to three days, and even longer if a live louse is found after a couple of days. A leave-in conditioner as well as the normal conditioner being left in could also make it easier – but it's still laborious.

PUBERTY AND TEENS

Puberty, leading up to the teens, is a time for rapid metabolic changes, with primary as well as secondary sexual characteristics being the most obvious developments. Primarily, there are changes in the internal reproductive processes, and external signs of these occurrences are manifested in the genitals in boys and in the breasts in girls. The hair, being a secondary sexual characteristic, also changes, not only on the scalp, but on the body as well. By the teens the scalp hair has reached its largest diameter and is at its thickest. Unfortunately, this is where the good news often ends.

The oil glands work overtime, the hair is usually worn longer and the hair often acquires an odd, almost rancid odour. 'You've got smelly hair' is the taunt given from one teenager to another. The one taunting may well have the odour themselves but can't smell it. Mothers bring their teenagers to see me to find out if anything is wrong. But it's not really an ailment: it is natural to produce oil and sweat, and the hormone surge and its continuation can result in extra production of these secretions. The cause of the odour is lack of hygiene – it's like body odour of the scalp. Body odour is cured by regular bathing, and smelly hair can similarly be removed by daily shampooing. Teenagers are notoriously sensitive to any negative remarks about them, so parents need to tread very carefully when trying to recommend something for smelly hair. It's really best not to draw attention to it, but instead treat them to an expensive, premium quality, nice smelling shampoo and conditioner as a gift, perhaps for doing something to help you. And say to them, 'These smell so nice that your boyfriend/girlfriend will love smelling you!' Or something to that effect. Daily washing is such an easy cure – it's just simple hygiene.

Without detracting from shampooing, teenage diets are not the best, and all the junk food with their high fat or sugary content can also effect the skin secretions adversely. However, this is really difficult to control, so you should try to counteract junk by giving them salads, vegetables and fruit at every possible occasion – if, indeed, they want to eat them when these foods are offered. Difficult, I know – I've been through it!

At about age eighteen the secretions will begin to slow, but by that time teenagers have usually become quite self-critical, even narcissistic, and will be taking much more notice of themselves anyway without any prompting.

I've not yet finished with adolescence. Added to everything else, it is the age when dandruff can rear its ugly head. And dandruff in the early teens is extremely common. But more about this in the relevant chapter – which, as it so happens, follows this.

10

Dandruff and Other Scalp Problems

DANDRUFF

The first mistake when dealing with dandruff is to associate it with 'dry scalp' or even dry skin when if fact it's mostly found in people with oily skin. The previous chapter discussing adolescents alludes to this time as when dandruff first appears. One of the reasons is that the sebaceous (oil) glands step up their oil production at puberty, giving greasier skin and scalp due to hormonal – mainly androgen (male hormones) – increase. It is also the age when stress increases and diets are at their worst. All of which effect scalp flaking.

Dandruff is the ultimate bad joke, a social stigma. You are made to believe that having white flakes on your collar or scratching your scalp will make you a social outcast, unable to make friends, influence people or even get a date. Yet dandruff strikes nearly everyone at one time or another.

The word dandruff is rather a loose one given to all types of scalp flaking, from common dandruff, be it loose or tight flakes, to a wickedly bothersome form of flakes that cling to the hair shaft as much as quarter of an inch (5mm) or more above the scalp and can cause hair loss. The commonest form of dandruff is known as pityriasis capitis simplex or pityriasis steatoides. If you have this, and most sufferers do, you may notice that it flares up under stress, although you may not always make the connection.

Dandruff occurs in this way: as you know, the skin all over your body is constantly being shed as a form of natural cell replacement,

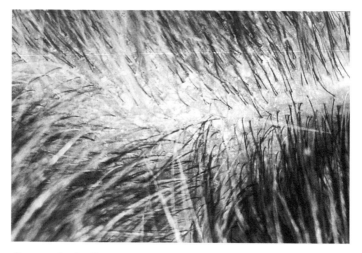

Common dandruff

which goes on internally as well as externally. Normally it goes unnoticed, the dead skin being washed away or rubbed off by our clothes. The skin shedding also occurs on our scalp, and this, too, should be unnoticed and washed away with shampooing. However, research indicates that metabolic changes can increase scalp skin shedding. Micro-organisms (bacteria, germs, though the main culprit is thought to be *pityrosporon ovale*) constantly inhabit the skin's surface. Your natural skin secretions such as sweat and sebum form a protective covering that keeps these bacteria dormant. Stress, hormonal changes and dietary misbehaviour (such as lots of salty, sugary or fatty foods) can cause the skin secretions to change adversely, lose their resistance to the ever-present bacteria, and as a consequence, the skin flora, as they are called, multiply, leading to an accelerated shedding of scalp skin – your 'dandruff flakes'. Contrary to what it seems and you may think, this is not dry scalp: the chances are the flakes are oily. The flakes absorb the sebum produced by your hair follicles, while a serum, which is also produced as a pre-inflammatory secretion, binds the flakes together, making rather tighter, stickier and larger flakes. It all sounds so horribly complicated but it isn't really.

SEBORROEIC DERMATITIS

This occurs if the skin becomes inflamed, even more serum is produced, making even larger flakes covering a reddening area of the scalp – primarily confined to the front area, below the forehead, behind the ears and the nape of the neck, as well as random patches over the scalp and even the eyebrows and nose area and centre of the chest. Either of these flakings or scalings is accompanied by itching – not always but usually. It has never ceased to amaze me that really heavy scales often cause less itching and scratching than the milder, lighter types – again, not always, but often enough to cause me to wonder.

Because of the apparent 'crustiness' of seborrhoeic dermatitis, the flakes are also thought to be dry. They're not: similarly to the milder form of dandruff, they are oily. The extra secretion of serum, which does dry up to a degree and feels tight, gives the impression of a dry scalp. It goes without saying that the more severe the flaking, the worse the hair will look. It can become dull, lank and limp.

Because the immediate reaction is to think the flakes are dry, oil is plonked on, rubbed in and the thinking is that the 'dry scalp' has gone. All it does, sadly, is to make the flakes greasier and more adherent, as well as resulting in greasy and lanker hair.

There is, furthermore, a question of susceptibility: it tends to run in families. There is no doubt, though, that fluctuations in the severity of flaking occur with stress; premenstrual stress in women, too, which also is connected to hormonal balances; certain foods, not necessarily the same ones for everybody, but more so with dairy products; and sometimes the type of shampoo you use.

Clearing common dandruff is easy. There are many effective anti-flaking, anti-itching shampoos to choose from that would work on most people. If the flakes are particularly nasty and tight or there is mild seborrhoeic dermatitis, there are some very good creams or scalp masques available. You can even ask your chemist or pharmacist to make a cream for you: 1 per cent each of sulphur and salicylic acid mixed in an oil-in-water emulsion can be very effective. Apply before shampooing in partings, massage it in, leave for ten to fifteen minutes, then wash off.

Alternatively, you can make your own anti-flaking scalp tonic by shaking together a mouthwash of your choice with an equal quantity of witch hazel. After rinsing off your shampoo and conditioner and towel drying your hair, sprinkle some of the mixture all over your scalp in partings, rub it in lightly with your fingertips and leave it on – you can additionally use whatever your normal styling aids are and blow dry it as usual. Contrary to popular thought, styling aids and blow dryers do *not* cause dandruff.

Using some or all of the above will clear up most forms of dandruff – if not, you may have one of the more serious forms of flaking described in the following paragraphs.

PSORIASIS

It seems that any bad scalp flaking is thought to be psoriasis by the lay public. Often they may be (erroneously) told by their doctor that they have psoriasis, when in fact it's just a form of heavy scaling or a type of seborrhoeic dermatitis.

Psoriasis is rarely found to be confined to the scalp alone, although the scalp can be severely affected by tenaciously adherent scales and underlying redness. The most common other parts of the body affected are the elbows and knees – and indeed this can be a diagnostic feature of the condition. It is odd, though, that even the worst cases of scalp psoriasis do not always cause itching.

Its cause still remains uncertain. Genetics, arthritic tendencies, food allergies, stress and long-standing infections have all been cited.

It can occur at any age, but it is most prevalent between twenty and thirty. Another strange feature is that psoriasis doesn't result in a large amount of hair loss. If the plaques of scale are very tight and of long duration, there may be a change in hair diameter together with an increased tendency to hair breakage. This is due to possible changes in hair structure, too, but I have not observed bald areas due to the condition itself. However, psoriasis is often confused with another very nasty and troubling scalp scaling called Pityriasis Amientacea, which can cause distinct hair loss.

Psoriasis often improves during the summer, which leads me to believe that the extra ultra-violet light helps – and ultra-violet light can be an effective treatment. Another point to remember about this is that stress factors are less during warm summer months and the hair is washed more often.

Treatment of psoriasis needs care and patience. At my clinics we often spend two hours gently removing the scales after they have been softened with creams containing coal tar, sulphur and salicylic acid under a warm steamer and infrared lamps. This can considerably alleviate it, but constant care needs to be taken over a long period of time.

PITYRIASIS AMIENTACEA

This can also be wickedly bothersome: it consists of tight scales in patches anywhere on the scalp. In time, these scales 'build up' on themselves, cling closely together and result in hard patches with matted hair at the roots. It can also, and often does, cause hair loss. But hair loss from it is usually reversible. The most common age, it seems, is between thirty-five and fifty.

It is not difficult to cure when correctly treated similarly to psoriasis. But I have already mentioned that diagnosing is sometimes difficult, as other scalp conditions can be confused with it.

NEURODERMATITIS

This is a hard, patchy scale most often confined to the upper nape of the neck. It can be maddeningly itchy, and scratching aggravates it by making it bleed. The persistent physical trauma of scratching can

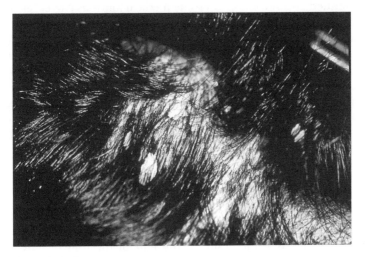

Pityriasis Amientacea

cause the flakes to become even harder. It is most common in middle-aged women, and as its name suggests, is associated with nerves and the nervous system. Treatment is similar to that of psoriasis.

CONTACT DERMATITIS

As its name implies, this is an inflammation of the scalp due to contact with an allergy-producing product, the most read-about being the severe reaction from hair colouring, which can occur in a very small percentage of those using them (see Chapter 12 on 'Hair Colouring'). But there are sometimes instances whereby a mild itching and flaking occurs if there is a sensitivity to a specific ingredient in one of the hair care products you use. This doesn't necessarily always occur, which leads me to believe that other factors are also involved, one of them being stress, another food and others a combination of what you use on your hair in the way of styling.

AIDS AND SCALP FLAKING

I have not yet seen any documentation on the prevalence of 'dandruff' in those people with AIDS. I have seen many HIV positive males and a few females. The first medical writings on AIDS were published around 1988, and some medical journals cite eczema as an early sign. Other symptoms may include premature greying, a flaky or dry skin and extra hair shedding. But heavy scalp flaking is not uncommon. Stress can also be a factor in these, and of course the stress involved in suffering from AIDS is huge. Also, as mentioned in Chapter 16 on 'Side Effects', AIDS drugs can cause hair fall and skin flaking. This chapter, though, would not have been complete without me mentioning the condition and its effect on the scalp and hair.

FOLLICULITIS

This is an inflammation of the hair follicle whereby a tiny pustule is formed at the hair follicle's opening. It can cause intense itching and tenderness – and result in the hair of the follicles affected being shed prematurely. Treatment with antiseptic creams or lotions, or sometimes an antibiotic, clears the condition. It is another one with sporadic flare-ups.

RINGWORM

Not often mentioned these days, although rare, it does occur, and should be borne in mind with pre-pubescent children. Also, the introduction of the antibiotic griseofulvin has almost wiped it out. Ringworm is a fungus infection and can result in scaly circular bald patches. It is easy to diagnose and the antibiotic works very rapidly.

ROSACEA

This often affects the scalp but is relatively easy to diagnose because the face and cheeks show signs of red blotches and scaly patches. The scalp almost always has some flaking and itching.

LICHEN SIMPLEX

These are small, round, flat and hard skin surfaces with an almost leathery look. It is very much alike to neurodermatitis, but the continual scratching and rubbing cause a 'lichenfication' – a thickening of the area that is constantly rubbed. Stress is thought to play a role in this, too. Salicylic acid cream together with sulphur and tar extract applied on a daily basis is beneficial. Alternatively, 1 per cent or 0.5 per cent of cortisone is often used.

You will have seen, yet again, how often stress affects scalp problems. Stress is, unfortunately, impossible to adequately control, but its effect should not be forgotten in any skin or hair complaint.

TICK BITES

Don't forget these in any scalp itching, particularly in the summer and autumn when ticks are at their height. The wonderful word 'no-see-ums' sums up ticks, and on warm, humid summer evenings they can certainly be bothersome. The only way to adequately deal with them is to wash your hair before going to bed.

Grey Hair

Unfortunately, grey hair is another ageing inevitability, and coping with it is sometimes difficult.

Despite the old adage 'better grey hair than no hair', your first grey hair doesn't do a lot for your morale. By the age of thirty most people have a few grey hairs, and by the age of fifty at least half of your hair will have turned grey. Some diseases may cause premature greying, for example diabetes, pernicious anaemia or thyroid problems. However, turning grey is also an inherited trait: if your parents went grey early, you will probably follow this pattern.

Dark-haired people are thought to turn grey earlier than others, but this is only because the grey hairs are more obvious. Fair-heads and blondes are the last to notice grey hair because of the subtler blending of white and blond. However, there is actually no such thing as a 'grey hair'. Grey is a combination of normally pigmented hairs interspersed with white ones. Hair turns white when the pigment cells responsible for colour stop being produced. These cells are formed at the base of the hair follicle, and the exact mechanism that causes the pigments to change is still something of a mystery.

Apart from genetics, nutritional and hormonal factors can affect hair colour, as can stress. We know that stress uses up vitamin B, and some studies have shown that certain B vitamins taken in large doses have begun to reverse the process of greying within three months. The hairs revert to white when the vitamins are stopped. Experiments with black rats (many years ago) showed that depriving them of the B vitamins turned their hair white. On reintroducing the vitamins, the hair regained its colour, an indication, perhaps, of the role of the B vitamins. But I haven't experienced this colour change with massive vitamin B doses.

Greying hair, like wrinkles, is associated with age, which is why there is such a huge trade in hair-colouring products. Contrary to popular belief, grey hair is not coarser; in fact, the chances are it will be finer, as everyone's hair gets finer with age. It may also become drier, because the oil glands likewise function less effectively as we get older, and this may give the impression of coarseness. Also, we often pull out our first few grey hairs in an attempt to remove the signs of ageing, and this constant pulling can distort the hair follicle, resulting in more crinkly hair, which gives the appearance of being coarser, too.

Grey hair should be handled in the same way as naturally pigmented hair. If you want to perm it, do so, but remember that perming can cause discoloration, turning the hair slightly yellow. Smoking can also lead to a yellowing of the hair. Using a blue rinse or even a blue-coloured shampoo can camouflage this yellow tinge. You should also remember that because grey hair lacks melanin (pigment), which in the skin protects against sun, its absence in the hair shaft could make it more vulnerable to sun damage as well.

At its best, grey hair can look wonderful, but if any type of hair needs frequent shampooing, it is grey hair, as it shows the dirt most of all. It is therefore advisable to wash and condition it daily.

There has been a lot of research into the gene that is responsible for turning off pigment production. The likelihood is that the gene will be isolated, its properties understood and eventually be modified to prevent greying. As with all gene manipulation, this is a long way off, so don't hold your breath! I wonder how the colour manufacturers view this? But it's not only those with grey hair who use colour – many others do just because they prefer a different look. The next chapter covers this aspect.

12

Hair Colouring

Everything You Need to Know

During the Introduction to this book I mentioned that I wrote a weekly series on hair colouring for the *Sunday Times* over a period of eight months – thirty-three weeks – during which time I saw thirty women and three men. I had the idea because of the enormous number of questions I had been asked over many years – which had been even more accelerated after I started writing for the *Sunday Times* 'Style' magazine.

Most of the fears were that colouring was going to make their hair fall out more. Or dry the hair or break it or affect their scalp.

I thought that I knew (more or less) what the effects of hair colouring were, but I wanted to run a series to prove my thoughts so that readers could know the truth and make their own choice.

It worked in this way: each week the beauty editor arranged for me to see a person of her choice who wanted their hair coloured. Some had already coloured their hair and wanted a change, others wanted to colour it for the first time. The three men were first-time colourers and oddly enough chose the most bizarre shades of all – perhaps because of repressed desires to use hair colouring (I have often said that men would like to colour their hair, but are wary of doing so for fear of being found out and thought of as a 'sissy').

However, I saw each person and made notes before they had their hair coloured at a salon of their choice or that of the beauty editor. However, some wanted to colour their hair at home and chose the method – semi-permanent usually, with the brand they fancied – and did indeed do it themselves. The different methods also added more credence.

I re-examined each one between four and seven days after having the colour.

Not one had extra hair fall. All of them, including the men, loved the result. None complained of extra dryness or breakage (I insisted they all followed the manufacturer's instructions and used the conditioner supplied with the pack). In fact, in most cases the hair was in better condition.

None of this surprised me – I pretty much knew it before we started. However, what *did* surprise me was that those with flaky and/or itchy scalps (some almost severe enough for me to withdraw them for the test) *all improved*! This was almost certainly due to the antiseptic properties the colouring agents contained, the mild keratalytic (softening and removing skin flakes) effects, and the thorough washing out that went along with the colouring process.

One of the myths in Chapter 27 on 'Hair Myths' is that hair colouring makes the hair fall. I say in the chapter that it doesn't.

Colouring your hair, of course, is entirely your own choice, and I am not advocating it to clear your scalp or help your hair. Hair colouring, I feel, does perhaps have an undeserved bad reputation.

Read on!

There is a pressure on all of us to remain youthful in our looks. A youthful appearance implies vigour, stamina, sex appeal and even optimism, although on occasions an unfavourable impression may be created, since youth can imply lack of experience or authority. Nonetheless, ageing is something most of us try to hide. Colouring your hair can give you a psychological boost, a sense of being a new and younger, more vital person. It is an easy way to change your personality or to discard part of an old life for a new one: changing hair colour when changing partners, for example.

Consequently, the hair-colouring market is enormous. It is estimated that almost 70 per cent of women and 12 per cent of men will colour their hair at some stage in their lives. The figures for men may be even higher, as many men are closet colourers and never admit to colouring their hair. They may steal their wife's products or use walnut oil or tea or coffee from the larder to make their own infusions to colour their hair. Some resort to mascara and many use progressive dyes, which change hair colour gradually over many applications, in a desperate attempt to disguise the fact that they have dyed their hair.

Why is there such a stigma attached to men who colour their hair? Women positively flaunt it. Perhaps it's because the practice is considered an unmasculine vanity. However, speaking as a man, and having advised thousands of men professionally, I am sure we are just as vain as women! And why shouldn't we be?

Apart from the desire to stay looking young, hair colour preferences are also influenced by fashion, usually following the film stars of the day. Hair was dyed red with Rita Hayworth, blonde with Marilyn Monroe, while many stars today have a sun-streaked look. In Cleopatra's day dark hair was the rage, and during the reign of Queen Elizabeth I ginger hair was popular.

However, whatever colour you decide on, you need to take precautions, as all colouring processes are potentially harmful if the instructions on the packaging are not followed.

COLOURING METHODS

First of all, I am not against any hair colouring method. In fact, the reverse is true: the psychological effects on changing hair colour far outweigh any potential physical damage to the hair.

There are many ways to colour hair and the choice of products is better now than ever before. The improvement in formulations give superior shades, and their safety is constantly monitored. Because of this, the so-called 'Natural' colour market has diminished; however, for whatever reason, many still use them for apparent feel-good or 'green' reasons.

'Natural' Colours

Henna, camomile, indigo and various other herbs have been in use for thousands of years. When the Pharaohs were buried, they often had their hair darkened to make them look young again. The Romans used pastes made of powder (talc) and various soaps derived from plants. Boiled and crushed walnuts, soot, burnt and charred ants' eggs, various berries and putrefied animal remains were used – all for the psychological boost of either masking white hairs or following the fashion of the times. Some years ago there was a huge leaning towards henna, not only as a colour, but as a panacea. It is emphatically not the latter and is only a poor substitute for the former. Henna gives unnatural shades of red which quickly fade, therefore encouraging multiple applications with an uneven distribution of colour from roots to ends. It can also turn orange in the sun or a ginger shade if permed. Camomile has also enjoyed a similar medicinal reputation; however, like that of henna, the reputation is somewhat unfounded. Camomile, though, can be a scalp soother for tenderness or itching. 'Natural' products are also discussed in Chapter 27 on 'Hair Myths'.

Colour Rinses or Temporary Colouring

These colours rest on the hairs' surface, are applied after each shampoo and last until the following shampoo; they used to be quite popular with the 'blue rinse brigade' to make yellowing-grey hair appear whiter. They still have their uses, particularly as a temporary method of covering grey between permanent colouring, but also to attain or improve an existing dye shade. The disadvantage of colour rinses is that they rub off onto pillows and can give a less than natural-looking shade. They also discolour the scalp, but this can be an advantage if the hair is thin, as it diminishes the contrast between the white scalp and the coloured hair. Another positive aspect of colour rinses is that they can reduce scalp shininess – if the scalp is very shiny, it will reflect more light and therefore draw more attention to it when the hair is thin. The main disadvantage, however, is that they discourage frequent shampooing because of the bother of re-applying the colour each time. Formulation of temporary colours are rather difficult because the 'dye' has to have what are apparently contradicting characteristics: they need to be relatively substantive (they need to cling firmly onto the hair), resistant to rain or perspiration, spread and cover evenly, yet still be easily removed by shampooing.

Semi-Permanent Colour

As the name suggests, these are longer lasting – up to about six weeks. They penetrate the outer cuticle of the hair, so resisting removal. The colours produced are more natural than the colour rinses described above, and semi-permanent colorants are also easier to use. Unlike permanent colours, they do not require pre-mixing but are used straight from the applicator, leading to the term 'direct dyes', as they are used directly from the bottle and do not need time to develop like the permanent dyes. Unlike the permanent dyes, they are applied to wet, washed hair, then the surplus rinsed off. The disadvantage, however, is that they fade with shampooing and exposure to air, leading to frequent reapplication. The ends of the hair therefore tend to get darker because they receive more applications than the roots. This is the reverse of what should occur: the ends should be lighter than the roots because of exposure to the air and sun. Therefore the overall appearance may be less than natural.

Some of the ingredients found in both colour rinses and semi-permanent colours are potentially sensitizing, so it is always advisable to do a patch test first by following the instructions on the packaging. This type of colouring is mostly used at home, and however inconvenient it may seem, the test should be done prior to each time it is applied. Sensitivities can be acquired for no apparent reason.

Permanent Dyes

These are often known as 'oxidation' dyes because an 'oxidizer' (for instance hydrogen peroxide) and ammonia are mixed with the colouring agent prior to application. Until the peroxide is added, the colour agent – in a separate bottle – is a clear liquid or whitish cream. The specific shade required is formed by the mixing of the second bottle containing the peroxide oxidizer. The formulation of permanent dyes is extremely complicated, and manufacturers go to great lengths to attain colour fastness and minimal disruption of the hairs' strength and elasticity. Added to all this, safety in use is a prime factor.

SENSITIVITIES, ALLERGIES AND CANCER RISKS

From time to time a truly scaremongering story emerges about hair colouring. One was when a woman had a violent allergic reaction and died of anaphylactic shock. The chances of this occurring are practically nil if a skin patch test is taken according to instructions. It is estimated that 4 in 1 million (1 in 250,000) are sensitive to hair dyes. It is probably more frequent, but the percentage is still small. The small percentage of risk tends to put people off the inconvenience of doing a 'patch test' whereby you need to wait a minimum of 24 hours to monitor any reaction. I can't emphasize sufficiently the importance of these tests for safe colouring. In addition, many think that once they have had a patch test they can continue colouring their hair without repeating it. Unfortunately, this is wrong. An allergy may develop between uses. Changes in stress, diet, medication or environment can all heighten the risk of acquiring a sensitivity. Use the patch test method before each colouring – and carefully follow instructions for it.

There is another drawback to patch testing: you go to your hair salon and suddenly decide that you want your hair coloured. The colourist can fit you in immediately because of a cancellation, otherwise you will have to wait another week. What do you do? Of course you grab the moment; 99 per cent (or more) of the time, all is well. But it is that very small risk that should make you rethink. The colourist, in all probability, wants the business and doesn't discourage you – *but* think again! All manufacturers put warnings on their labels, now more prominent than ever. Safety is their principal and essential concern. Heed them.

Cancer

The latest scare is that of colourings causing bladder cancer. One of the first reports on the links between hair dyes and bladder cancer was over twenty years ago. Another scare was about five years ago, and another one more recently. None of the studies could be sufficiently substantiated, although colour manufacturers modified some formulations.

Each study used similar methods: the hair of mice was shaved daily and the colour applied to the skin afterwards. After three months (about 100 applications) most of the mice developed bladder cancer. To base the resultant scaremongering on these results appears to be unreasonable and even unjust: shaving the skin sensitizes and increases absorption rates, and the constant daily application would have a greater effect than occasional use. The equivalent in a human, averaging six weeks between dyes, is 600 weeks, or twelve years. But the scalp (obviously) is not shaved and sensitized, nor does the build-up effect of daily applications occur.

It has not been made clear whether there have been double blind tests either, comparing similar age groups of those using dyes long term and those who are not for twelve years. In that time as a person gets older, the cancer risks increase anyway.

Some other studies have detected no increased risk of bladder cancer. One that examined nearly 600 women followed by the American Cancer Society and 120,000 by Harvard University, plus a study in Italy, concluded that, 'the overall evidence excluded any appreciable and measurable risk of bladder cancer from personal use of hair dyes'.

It is important to remember the huge psychological boost that hair colour gives, and people would do it even if it were harmful – which as yet, if ever, hasn't been proven.

BLEACHING AND HAIR LIGHTENING

These do not add but remove colour. Their oxidizing effect decolourizes the pigment in the hair shaft and lightens the colour. If a bleach is left on long enough, it will turn the hair almost white! Hydrogen peroxide and ammonia are the most commonly used bleaching ingredients, although many products claim to contain no peroxide, in which case another oxidizing ingredient will have been used that will have a similar effect. *All* bleaches have a damaging effect on the hair's protein structure, making the hair dry, brittle and inelastic, and often leading to breakage. The hair also becomes more porous and more vulnerable to other chemical processes such as permanent wave solutions in curling or straightening. There is also a greater vulnerability to sun damage, swim damage and wind damage. Bleaching also softens the skin, so it is important not to rub the scalp vigorously when washing out the bleach.

It is impossible to make the hair a lighter shade without the help of a bleaching agent – and all of them are called 'oxidizing agents' (the main one being hydrogen peroxide, as stated). However, used alone it is not stable, and very slow in lightening the hair. To hasten its effect it needs to be mixed with an alkaline solution just prior to application – the most common being ammonia. Peroxide and ammonia on their own are very runny and impossible to control in just one area – it would run onto already bleached parts. Because of this, bleaches are made into creams with oils and waxes (emulsions), and the ammonia is added before applying to the hair.

It is usually not necessary to have a skin sensitivity test for bleaches, but bleaching agents are rarely used on their own because they do not give natural shades. They result in rather brassy-looking straw-like hair, so various colour agents are added to reduce brassiness and give the shade required.

Of all the colouring methods, bleach is potentially the most damaging, and therefore should ideally be done professionally. If bleaching your own hair, exercise great caution: read and re-read the instructions carefully.

Highlighting, Streaking and Frosting

These are all similar procedures. Small tufts of hair are bleached either by pulling through a cap pierced with holes or by carefully separating them, then applying the bleach and wrapping the hairs in foil. It is a very effective way of blending grey hair or giving your hair a sun-streaked, outdoor look. Only a portion of the hair is bleached and, moreover, the colour lasts longer because of the blending and is thus used less often, making this one of the safer colouring methods. However, overlapping previously bleached tufts can be a problem.

Single or Double Processing?

It is not possible to get an exact shade or tone by bleaching alone. Modern methods of colouring are usually done in a single process. In the early days two processes were given. As previously mentioned, leaving pure bleach on the hair will give a yellowish-red tone, so most bleaching products also contain a colorant to counteract this effect. Therefore all bleaching products are, in a way, double processes in a single application.

A double process was to lighten the hair first with a bleaching agent, rinse it off and then use a dye to reach the colour required. A single process will combine these two procedures; although more difficult to formulate, such products are actually easier to use. However, it is debatable as to whether a single process is better for the hair than two applications: the same chemical and physical actions occur either way. Of course, the timesaving aspect is obvious.

Taking Care of Coloured Hair

Having your hair coloured in a salon will certainly involve some conditioning treatment. If you colour your hair at home, the package will contain an efficient conditioner, too. All very necessary.

Any hair that has undergone dyeing is vulnerable to damage; the degree to which damage is done, however, is dependent on the amount of colour change. For instance, going from a dark to a light shade is the most dangerous because the colouring (bleaching) agent is stronger or left on for longer. Obviously the frequency with which hair is dyed is a major factor in the amount of damage sustained. Any chemical process reduces the hair's elasticity (stretchability) and increases the prospect of hair breakage. Apart from the after colour conditioning treatment, use a deep conditioner prior to shampooing your hair a couple of days before and after colouring. Such conditioning treatments should also be used weekly if the hair is bleached.

It is similarly important to condition *after* every shampoo, as this will eliminate tangles and smooth the hair cuticles raised by the alkaline solutions. The heavier, more moisturizing types of products should be chosen, irrespective of the possibility of causing fine hair to turn limp. Any limpness can be counteracted by styling aids. There are many treatment products available as pre-shampoo remoisturizers. If you wish to make your own, whisk in a blender:

2 eggs
1 tbsp of any thick, off-the-shelf conditioner
½oz castor oil
1 ripe avocado
1oz full cream milk

Refrigerate overnight. Apply the mixture to the hair in sections, working it into the hair with your fingers, particularly at the ends. Cover the hair with a damp, warm towel or cap and, if possible, leave in overnight. Shampoo and condition as usual.

It is important to handle your hair gently: hard brushing, rubbing too hard with a towel when drying, keeping the hairdryer on for too long, having it too hot, pulling too hard – all should be avoided.

CHOOSING YOUR COLOUR

The array of colours displayed in stores is quite mind boggling and, to say the least, confusing. Undoubtedly, it's best to have your hair coloured in a salon. The colourist will be more knowledgeable than you, have more experience, apply the colour more uniformly and, very importantly, be able to monitor the action. But expense or timing comes into it, and many do not want to spend the money or are unable to find the time to fit in with the colourist.

It is difficult to understand the logic of hair colour manufacturers: they spend a fortune on training hairdressers how to use the colouring product, but I have yet to see a colour advisor in shops that sell hair colours, although it is commonplace to have beauty advisors to help choose make-up. Hair, as I have so often mentioned, has a psychological impact greater than any other – and hair colour is part of that. The average consumer is daunted by choice when entering the colour section of a store. Not only that, many are unsure which colour would best suit them.

Most manufacturers have consumer advisory services that are most helpful, but it doesn't make up for a colour expert being able to see you in person. There are probably reasons for this personal service not being available, but I can't see what they are.

All colour companies have excellent research facilities and constant safety measures in place. Hair colours now are better than ever before. The packaging for home use contains first-class conditioning agents to use with or after the colour process; instructions for use are clear and concise; and they even supply gloves! Why not have the ultimate personal advice available?

13

Perming and Straightening

Following on from hair colouring and its psychological and physical effects, perming and straightening can be another potential hazard – but it shouldn't be.

PERMING

Fashions come and go, and the 'fashion' of hair perming is not as popular now as it once was. The main reason, it seems, is that the curly look, most fashionable perhaps in the late 1970s, is at present considered passé. This is not to say that it won't eventually return. Another reason is hair styling products. It is only during the past ten to fifteen years that new ingredients have allowed the formulation of styling products that give the hair 'body' and apparently more thickness and control. One of the prime purposes of 'perms' in women over forty, when the hair loses body and volume, was to mask its thinning by making it wavy or curly and to swell the hair strands so that the hair looked and felt thicker. Nowadays, women in their fifties and sixties are more likely to have their hair permed – and if the hair is straight and limp, younger women may also be tempted by what are termed 'body waves'.

You may be surprised to hear that, historically, hair waving was used in the mid-seventeenth century to curl wigs. The hair was rolled on cylinder-shaped baked clay and heated with hot water for many hours and then allowed to dry.

The underlying principle of waving hair is its elasticity. When hair is wet, it stretches and swells – in a way becomes deformed – and its disulphide bonds are disrupted. Yet the hair goes back to its original shape as it dries. If the hair is rolled up before it dries, it will dry into the shape it is put, i.e. waves or curls. Heat accelerates this. The shape the hair dries into will remain until it is wet or dampened or absorbs atmospheric moisture. 'Permanent' waves carried this a stage further by using chemicals instead of water. At first this was done by applying heat to alkaline chemicals, then in the 1940s 'cold waves' were introduced, whereby the hair was wetted with the waving solution, rolled up (the size of the curls depending on the roller size), left to process for a specified time, then 'fixed' in its curly shape by a 'neutralizer' lotion.

This method revolutionized perming by its ease and relative comfort. It reached its peak by the marketing of 'home perms', enabling the whole process to be done by the individual herself.

The market in home perms now is much smaller, the preference being (if required) to have it done in a salon. Because the solutions used are strongly alkaline, there is the possibility of severe damage unless great care is taken. The common ingredients used are ammonium thioglycollate to 'reduce' the bonds, and an oxidizing agent such as hydrogen peroxide to 'fix' the shape.

Skin is a similar structure to hair, so the scalp may become tender or a little sore after all the waving solutions are washed out.

The damage to hair is minimal when applied correctly. However, problems can occur quite easily by leaving the solutions on the hair for too long, rolling too tightly or failing to thoroughly neutralize.

STRAIGHTENING

This is a very similar procedure to perming, but instead of waving straight hair, you straighten wavy hair. Straightening is potentially more damaging: the solution is put on at scalp level, the hair is gradually pulled straight with a special comb, and when sufficiently straight it is 'fixed' in this shape. It is most commonly used on Black hair, and some of the worst cases of hair breakage occur unless great care is taken. Straightening is done more often than perming – approximately every six to eight weeks – so the risk of overlapping previous processing is considerable. It is this overlapping that causes most problems. See also Chapter 3 on 'The Ethnic Behaviour of Hair'.

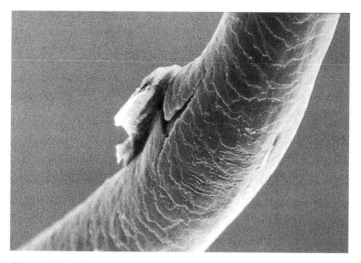

Fractured hair from too tight perming

It is always best to have straightening done by a professional who can carefully monitor the process.

Remember that the temperature of the room can increase the speed of chemical reactions, working faster on a hot day than on a cold day, something your hair stylist should also bear in mind. Therefore careful monitoring is essential *every* time your hair is permed – another reason for professional care.

It is important to deep-condition your hair twice a week for two weeks prior to either process. There are some excellent deep-conditioning products available, and it is best to use one of them rather than attempt to make your own. However, if you prefer it, I recommend the following recipe. Whisk together:

1oz of any heavy-conditioning cream
2 eggs
1oz of a light vegetable oil

Apply over the hair in one-inch partings, paying particular attention to the ends. Lightly rub the mixture into the ends between your thumb and finger tips. Leave under a bathing cap for up to half an hour, then shampoo and condition as usual. After perming, wait a few days, then use the mixture again.

Never perm (or straighten) your hair on the same day as colouring it. It is best to leave a week in between, perming first and then colouring a week later. For the best results, deep-condition your hair between perming and colouring.

Avoid perming if the skin on your scalp is inflamed or broken. If the scalp becomes inflamed or irritated after perming, apply a solution of cold milk and water in equal parts, which should help to soothe it. If the condition persists, you should really consult a dermatologist.

It is important to remember that hair grows half an inch (1.25cm) a month, so think about the potential overlapping problems.

Perming virgin hair seldom results in disaster; however, perming previously permed hair can do a great deal of damage – I have seen ends of hair that look and feel like Brillo. A good way to avoid this is to protect the ends with a heavy fat such as unsalted butter before the perm solution is applied. 'Root perms', whereby only the roots or unpermed part of the hair are permed, attempt to address this problem, but this is a rather troublesome procedure, as the overlapping of already permed hair is difficult to avoid and the scalp often suffers as a result.

As I have already stated, I am not attempting to put you off perming – it can be an immense boost to your morale. I am just pointing out the dangers. After all, this section *is* to tell you about perming!

14

Styling Your Hair Safely

Part of this chapter should include the previous two chapters – 'Colouring' and 'Perming and Straightening' – which are, in a way, styling procedures. But the following is how to achieve the finished product, so to speak.

To have your hair looking the way you want often involves potentially damaging procedures. But it is just as easy to do these correctly as incorrectly. And it is important not to undo the good work of shampooing and conditioning.

HOW TO DRY YOUR HAIR FAST WITHOUT DRYING IT OUT

Now that you have correctly washed and conditioned your hair, you will probably want to dry it. The secret of safe drying is good timing, and every second counts. The ideal way to dry your hair is to pat it with a towel and then let it dry naturally. This is fine as long as you don't mind getting up at 5 a.m. every day or how it looks when dry.

The obvious alternative is to use a dryer, but you have probably heard that all dryers dry your hair out and split the ends. Furthermore, you have probably blamed the dryer for dandruff, hair fall and an itchy scalp. The poor hairdryer! It has a much maligned and completely undeserved reputation. As with so many things in life, it's not what you do but the way in which you do it that matters, or, in the case of hair drying, it's not what you use but the way you use it.

Moisture is as important to the hair as it is to the skin. It is moisture, not oil, that keeps the hair soft and resilient. Overuse of a hairdryer can rob the hair of this precious moisture, leaving it dry, dull and brittle. The easiest, most popular way to dry hair is with a hand-held blowdryer, and once you know how to use it, you can do it both quickly and safely. Try to follow these few, simple steps.

Towel Drying

After showering, resist the temptation to vigorously rub your head with a towel, as this can break your hair and possibly pull it out. Instead, press your hair with a towel to remove excess moisture, then carefully ease out any tangles with a wide-toothed comb, starting at the ends.

Choosing the Right Hairdryer

It should have separate controls for temperature and speed. Anything stronger than 1200 watts is unnecessary. Special diffuser attachments that fit over the nozzle spread the heat over a wider area. The wider the attachment, the better the heat is diffused. However, for fast drying don't use an attachment.

Using the Hairdryer

Hold the dryer about 6 inches away. Dry the back and sides of your head first, and work towards the crown and front. Start on a high speed and high temperature, and then, as the hair begins to dry, gradually reduce the heat. If you use a brush for styling, choose one made of soft, pliable plastic and use it gently, as a brush can do more damage than a hairdryer.

Finishing Off

When the hair is almost dry, turn down the heat and reduce the speed. Check the hair constantly. It is at this point that damage is most likely to occur, so care needs to be taken. It is odd that to counteract damage, many people allow their hair to dry naturally until damp and then blow dry to finish it off – and finish it off they might! Blow drying hair from wet to damp does no damage, but drying from damp to dry can be hazardous. Ideally, the hair *should* be left damp, but if you need your hair absolutely dry, it is vital to stop blow drying at the right time. That extra few seconds can dry out the moisture content in the hair cells and lead to brittleness, dullness, breakage and split ends.

Adding Volume

If you have limp, thin or straight hair, as you finish drying, bend over and, still using the hairdryer, let your hair hang down towards the floor. Gently brush or comb your hair in this direction with the dryer following behind. This gives the hair more lift and bounce, decreases the likelihood of tangles, improves scalp circulation and generally increases volume and body (see also p.26 on 'Hair Body').

ROLLERS

Most people use rollers at one time or another to enhance their hairstyle, to give it more curl or wave, to control curls and frizz, to give it more body or lift, or to make it smooth.

Choosing rollers

Look for smooth or foam-covered rollers without spikes and, preferably, without a Velcro-like covering. Such rollers can not only tangle the hair, but can also be impossible to remove without breaking off some hair.

Do not roll the hair too tightly: this is a frequent cause of hair breakage and hair loss. People with fine, limp hair often believe that a style will last longer the tighter the hair is rolled. This may be marginally true, but it creates a vicious circle, as the tighter the rollers, the more likely it is that hair will be pulled out and broken, causing the hair to thin and, in turn, leading to the use of even tighter rollers in an attempt to disguise the thinning.

And of course never go to sleep with rollers in your hair, as this will almost certainly damage it and lead to hair loss. Rubbing hair between rollers and pillow as you change position during the night will pull on the hair roots and can also result in lethal tangling.

CURLERS

These are similar to rollers but are not often used these days, except in permanent wave kits.

If you are tempted, the old-fashioned curlers consisting of felt-wrapped pliable wire are the best. The hair is wrapped round one end and the other end is twisted back over to keep it in place.

To use the modern type of curlers the hair is wrapped round the centre and then held in place with a clip. Be careful that the clip is not too tight.

Whether using rollers or curlers, always remember not to roll too tightly, and do not over-dry with a hairdryer.

HEATED ROLLERS

Unlike curlers, these are becoming more popular. They are convenient and quick to use and are a great morale booster. They should be used after shampooing or to freshen up a style on dry hair. However, just because they are easy to use, do not overuse them, as this can result in dried and split hair. Following the correct procedures will minimize the risks.

Choose steam-producing, thermostatically controlled rollers.

It's best to use heated rollers after shampooing and conditioning the hair. If you need to use them unexpectedly between shampoos, protect the ends of the hair with a little tissue paper before putting in the rollers.

Heated rollers tend to be heavier and bulkier, so take care not to leave them in for too long.

As with all other curling methods, do not roll the hair too tightly.

HOT IRONS

If handled incorrectly, hot irons are a potential danger to hair, although if they are used with care, the damage they cause is minimal. There are two kinds of hot irons: one for curling hair and the other for straightening. Both types can be bought with a thermostatic control, but to ensure they do their job properly, make sure they are sufficiently heated. The heat required to temporarily realign the shape of the hair is considerable.

For irons to work effectively the hair should be fairly dry; in this way the natural moisture content of the hair is used to create a new style. However, if care is not taken, you can make your hair brittle.

Steam-producing irons are less likely to dry out the hair, as these provide moisture; Teflon-coated irons are best.

Hot Irons develops a residue from the impurities in water (distilled water should be used) and from scorched hair cells. As this is unavoidable, all irons will eventually need to be replaced, otherwise they will stick to the hair and cause problems. Do not be mean about this – throw them away as soon as 'stickiness' occurs.

Do not leave the iron on the hair for too long and do not pull excessively on the hair to straighten or curl. Also, try not to go too near to the scalp – burns are painful and can become infected.

HOT COMBS

Fortunately, hot combs are less popular now. They are mainly used to straighten tightly curled hair, particularly Black hair. To soften the hair a hot pressing oil is applied and a hot comb repeatedly pulled through the hair until it is straight. Hot combs can be difficult to control, and unless the utmost care is taken, severe breakage can result.

PINS AND CLIPS (AND SORE SCALPS)

If you are wondering why your hair is damaged or your scalp is sore, pins and clips may be the culprits.

Do not go to sleep with pins and clips in your hair, as the metal cuts into the hair shaft and the scalp.

If you are using them for curling, be careful when drying your hair. The heat of the dryer warms the metal, which can then damage the hair and scalp. The metal retains heat even after the dryer is removed, so you should move the dryer rapidly over your head in order to avoid over-heating any one area.

If you use a hood dryer, remove it frequently to allow the hair and scalp to cool.

ELASTIC BANDS AND BARRETTES (CLASPS)

Bands and barrettes are normally used to keep hair off the face, but barrettes are often used to add hair, like in a chignon, which adds false hair to that already there. Usually the hair is pinned at the crown to add a ponytail or to mask a flattening on the top of the head and give extra height. They are very effective but they can also be lethal, many times causing bald areas of traction alopecia. Great

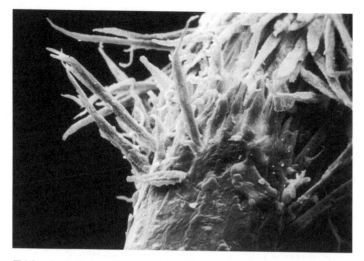

Trichorrhexis Nodosa (due to a tight elastic band)

care needs to be taken to avoid this. They should not be attached tightly to hair that has been pulled taught away from the scalp. Nor should they be slept in, as the metal clip will rub on the scalp, causing a sore and the hair can be rubbed away too.

Choose your barrette carefully. Inspect the metal edges for sharpness, and, as an added protection, wrap a thin strip of tissue or tape round the grip.

Elastic bands are most common of all. Normally used to put hair into a pigtail, if too tight, they cut into the hair shafts, resulting in Trichorrbexis Nodosa – a breakage of the hair, which when viewed under the microscope looks like two shaving brushes pressed together.

Also, pulling the hair too tightly back from the forehead can lead to a traction hair loss all along the front hairline and temples, or at least to a severe breakage in these areas. Young girls are most at risk – and, of course, ballet dancers, who also tend to have a degree of traction loss along the parting.

The worst culprits are the uncovered elastic band repeatedly twisted around the hair. When it is removed, it also removes some of the hair. Use a thick, fabric-coated band instead and smear a little conditioner along it for added protection.

15

Your Health and Your Hair

Most of you at one time or another have connected the behaviour of your hair with the way you feel: the state of your health, the degree of stress or worry, sleep patterns, pregnancies (in both sexes it may surprise you to know), menstrual cycle, short- or long-term illnesses, fevers and, very importantly, the drugs, vitamins and minerals you take to counteract them all (see Chapter 16 on 'Drug Side Effects'). Every one of them can effect your hair.

I have repeatedly said, for example, that there is always a reason for hair falling or thinning (not necessarily the same) – and when the reason is found, more often than not you can do something about it.

Hair is an incredibly sensitive barometer of your body; it is also a curious dichotomy. The rapidity with which hair cells are produced is second only to that of the fastest cell reproducer in your body, bone marrow.

But unlike bone marrow, hair is non-essential tissue; you can easily live without it, however much you need it psychologically. Your body metabolism aims to keep the essential tissues functioning first and foremost, and although hair-cell reproduction is only just behind that of bone marrow, the hair doesn't stand a chance of competing with this or other body-essential tissues for the necessary elements needed to maintain health.

However, the combination of hair-cell proliferation and your body's inclination to ignore its needs mean that hair is usually the first to suffer from any bodily upset and the last to benefit from an improvement. Indeed, your hair can forewarn you even when there are no other symptoms of illness. In Chapter 2 on 'Is Your Hair

Dead or Alive?' I discussed the remarkable properties of hair; this is another example of those properties.

At some stage we have all experienced what seem to be inexplicable variations in the way our hair looks and feels. Some of these are due to the products that have been used on it, the way in which they have been used, humidity levels or how we have styled it. But women also notice fluctuations at different stages of their monthly cycles, hair often being at its most lifeless just before menstruation.

None of these examples are as important as the hair's reaction to illness and, consequently, its invaluable use as a diagnostic tool. A sudden hair fall or hair not as thick as it was often indicates an underlying metabolic dysfunction or an illness. The most typical examples of conditions that affect hair are anaemia, thyroid dysfunction, hormonal disturbances and nutritional inadequacies. But in each case unless other symptoms are present, the sufferer is unlikely to be aware that his or her hair problems are due to any of them.

Other overlooked reasons for hair trouble are the effects of fever, accidents, operations or even pregnancy. Hair symptoms do not necessarily coincide with poor health – it can sometimes be as much as several months later that the effects on the hair become noticeable, by which time you may not connect the two events. A classic example of this is when the hair falls out two to three months after having a baby. Similarly, the trauma of an operation may not affect the hair for two to three months. It is interesting to note that although postoperative hair loss is still common, it occurs less frequently than it used to. The modern practice of getting the patient out of bed the next day leads to faster recovery and less hospital 'blues'.

Illness, operations, stress, shock, fever and metabolic trauma are all likely to affect the hair. It is important to realize this, as so often a hair-loss problem is dismissed by doctors as 'genetic' when this may not be the case at all.

Stress can be a considerable factor – and a question I am often asked is whether stress can affect hair loss. It can and often does. Stress can lead to the production of more adrenaline, which can be converted into cholesterol, which in turn could result in testosterone increases. Testosterone is a male hormone that when converted into di-hydrotestosterone can cause hair to thin.

The complexity of your hair's reactions to internal conditions cannot be underestimated, and I shall be discussing in more detail different aspects of your physical health and its affect on the condition of your hair.

SOME OTHER METABOLIC CAUSES
OF HAIR LOSS

You will have already realized that hormonal levels are important in maintaining your hair. There are other reasons, though, and they are aspects that should be borne in mind. One of them is iron levels. And although it is more commonly found in women, men can also be affected.

Anaemia

The incidence of anaemia in menstruating women is severely under-estimated, but even more so is the incidence of low iron levels, which is not necessarily the same thing. Anaemia is measured by haemo-globin, and is probably the most commonly measured constituent in a blood test. It measures red blood cells, the normal reference range being approximately 11.5–15.5 depending on the testing laboratory. Any reading below 0.5 higher than the low point (i.e. if 11.5 is lowest, anything below 12.0) could be a factor in hair thinning.

However, haemoglobin is only one of many iron tests; another is ferritin. Serum ferritin is a good indicator of available iron stores in the body. Decreases in ferritin levels, even if the haemoglobin is normal, can effect hair follicle function. The average reference ranges of ferritin are 15–170 (again, it varies with each laboratory). Recently, it has been established that anything below 27 in women is question-able as far as iron deficiency anaemia is concerned. However, for optimum hair follicle function, ferritin should be at a minimum of 70.

Many women go to their doctor for blood tests, anaemia being the most common, because most women suspect that anaemia can affect their hair – and although they would have a 'full blood count', ferritin is rarely included. It would not be considered relevant by your doctor. But it certainly is relevant, and iron medication from your doctor can prove to be extremely beneficial. It takes a long time to increase ferritin levels, perhaps as much as six months or more, so you don't get an immediate effect on your hair. However, as your fer-ritin increases, your hair will progressively benefit.

Iron is a mineral, and although it is one of the most important for your hair, there are others to be considered, such as zinc, mag-nesium and copper. The interaction between iron, zinc, copper and magnesium is complicated, and a low or high level of any could be a factor. Taking a well formulated mineral supplement could be helpful, irrespective of suspecting an imbalance.

Thyroid

The thyroid gland is crucial in maintaining the body's metabolism by controlling the production of proteins and tissue utilization of oxygen, thus affecting the hair follicles.

Understanding thyroid function and its effect on hair growth is very complicated, and I do not want to tempt you to blame a thyroid dysfunction for your hair fall or thinning hair. On the other hand, it may be useful for you or your doctor to realize that there is a possibility of having thyroid readings in the normal reference range but it still having an effect on your hair. That is, as with many blood test results, low normals or high normals can be one of the triggers.

Hypothyroid (low) or hyperthyroid (high) definitely affects hair adversely, but these are easily diagnosed by low or high thyroid testing levels. It is the ones on the cusp that sometimes need a mild degree of medication, but it is only available on prescription. However, your doctor may be reluctant to prescribe it if you are in the normal reference ranges.

A further complication is that thyroid production can be affected by other conditions: drugs, oral contraceptives, pregnancy and menopause for example. Long-standing hypothyroids may result in anaemia; people from developing countries may suffer from low iodine intake, which effects the thyroid and therefore the hair.

Two quite common thyroid diseases are Hashimoto's (hypo) and Grave's (hyper). Either of these would have other symptoms apart from hair loss. The high thyroids, for example, may have high blood pressure, a rapid heartbeat, increased sweating, insomnia, slightly protruding eyes and weight loss in spite of increased appetite. The low thyroids may experience, amongst other things, a slower pulse, hoarser voice, intolerance to cold, weight gain, thinner and dryer hair and loss of some eyebrow hair. If you begin to notice any of these, it would be as well to check with your doctor.

Almost without exception, women in particular will have had their thyroid checked before coming to see me for a hair problem – many of them having mild symptoms as mentioned, but still just in the normal range where medication is deemed unnecessary. Hair sensitive or hair sympathetic doctors seem in the minority, and as with blood tests and measurements for iron levels, thyroid measurements are accepted without due regard to their effect on the hair.

16

Drug Side Effects

It seems sensible to follow the last chapter on 'Your Health and Your Hair' with the way that drugs used to improve or maintain your health can affect your hair.

I have already discussed thyroid drugs whereby too much or too little can result in hair fall, hair brittleness, dryness and dullness. Also how iron supplements are needed to control iron levels. However, it seems strange that one of the most commonly overlooked reasons for hair or scalp misbehaviour is medications, drugs and even vitamin or mineral supplements. Unfortunately, in the case of life-threatening illness or reduction in the quality of life, the taking of drugs is inevitable even though they may lead to hair problems. And it is well to remember that often the effects of drugs on the hair are not immediate.

CHEMOTHERAPY

I hope I am not being seen as morbid to have chemotherapy as the first drug side effect. It is likely that everyone knows a person who has undergone the trauma of being diagnosed for cancer and having to be treated by chemotherapy – and it is common knowledge that one of its side effects can be hair loss. The disease, so distressing in itself, gives further distress and anxiety when one of the most upsetting side effects of treatment is loss of hair. In my practice hardly a day goes by without a reference or enquiry on it. I have had many women consult me prior to their chemotherapy about what they can do to avoid their hair coming out. And there was a time when it could not be avoided at all, which sometimes resulted in refusal to have chemotherapy for fear of going bald. It was only by means of extraordinary persuasion, making them believe that whatever hair fell out would regrow again, that they finally accepted the treatment.

However, the last two to three years has shown that the amount of hair fall can be contained. This is done by tightly bandaging ice packs around the head, inhibiting the flow of the chemical therapy around the head and thus inhibiting the flow of the chemical therapy to the scalp hair follicle capillaries. Some hair may still fall out, but not to the extent of almost baldness.

Although I strongly reiterate that complete regrowth of whatever is lost will occur, it is still difficult to initially convince the person to accept it. But, it *always* grows back. An odd feature of the regrowth may be that occasionally the hair grows back wavy when previously it had been straight, or vice versa. The point is it *does* grow back.

OTHER DRUGS WITH SIDE EFFECTS

I have discussed on previous pages the side effects of oral contraceptives and Hormone Replacement Therapy, some being better than others for your hair, so these chapters should also be referred to.

The complication of any drug is that by means of other metabolically normal functions, they may not have the same effect on everybody. One of these is aspirin. It is possible that long-term use of aspirin can lower haemoglobin levels. Antibiotics can do so as well.

This is also true of the group of drugs used to treat cardiovascular disease such as hypertension, or lipid (fats and cholesterol) regulators. Most of them can cause an extra hair shedding. Again, what may cause hair shedding on one person may not do so on another. Also, there are different classes of drugs used for similar purposes, and if one seems to increase hair fall, ask your doctor to try another. I want to stress that the incidence of hair fall problems from some of these drugs may be very small, but it is a factor to be borne in mind.

The most commonly prescribed drugs for hypertension and cholesterol control may be known by different names in the UK and USA. They are as follows (UK name followed by US name if different), in alphabetical order:

Accupro – Accupril
Accuretic
Acepril – Capoten
Adalat – Procardia
Alcoril
Aldoclor
Amias – Atacand
Angilol – Inderal
Arythmol – Rythmol
Atenix – Tenormin
Atromis
Betagan
Betaxon
Betimol
Blocadren
Cardura
Clorpres
Corgaretic – Corgard
Corzide
Cosopt – Timolide
Covera
Cozaar – Nyzaar
Diovah
Diuril
Dixarit – Catapres
Duraclon
Efexor – Effexor
Elmiron
Emcor – Zebeta
Enalaprila
Esidrex – Hydrodiur
Genotropi
Hep Flush – Heparin
Innozide – Vaseretic
Istin – Norvasc
Kerlone – Betoptics
Lexxel
Lipantil – Tricor
Lipitor
Lipobay – Baycol
Lipostat – Pravachol

Lopid
Lotensin
Marvan – Coumadin
Mexitil
Meyacor
Midamor
Nypovase – Minipress
Perdix – Uniretic
Sectral
Serostim
Sotacor – Batapace
Tambocor
Tarka
Tenex
Tenif – Tenoretic
Tonocard
Ucardic – Coreg
Zestoretic
Zestril
Ziac & Zocor

Many other drugs may have hair side effects. The following is a list together with what they are prescribed for. The UK name comes first and the US name second (if it is different), in alphabetical order:

Abelcet	Amphotec	Fungal infections
Accutane		For severe acne
Acitac	Tagamet	Duodenal ulcer, gastritis
Aggrenox		Reduces the risk of strokes
Alopral	Lopurin	Anti-gout
Aricept		Mild dementia of the Alzheimer type
Arthrosin	Anaprox	Anti-inflammatory and analgesic
Arthrotel		Analgesic and anti-inflammatory
Atrovent		Asthma and bronchitis
Betacap	Luxiq	Itching and anti-inflammation on skin
Brufen (Ibuprofen)	Motrin	Anti-inflammatory and analgesic

Casodex		Immunosuppressant for prostate cancer
Celance	Permax	Parkinson's disease
Cerubidine		Leukaemia
Ciproxin	Cipro HC	Antibacterial
Clarityn	Claritin	Antihistamine
Clinoril		Analgesic and anti-inflammatory
Colazide	Colazal	Colitis
Combivir		Antiviral HIV
Comvax		Hepatitis
Concordin	Vivactil	Antidepressant
Crixivan		Antiviral HIV
Cytotec		Gastritis
Dermovate	Temovate	Anti-inflammatory
Diclozip	Cataflah	Antidepressant
Diflucan		Anti-fungal
Dipentum		Colitis
Duovent	Combivent	Asthma and bronchial
Efexor	Effexor	Antidepressant
Engerix B		Hepatitis B vaccine
Epivir		Antiviral HIV
Erwinase	Oncaspar	Immunosuppressant
Exirel	Maxair	Anti-asthma
Famotidine	Pepcid	Gastro-intestinal
Flaverin	Luvox	Obsessive Compulsive Disorder
Flexeril		Muscle relaxant
Flexin	Indocin	Anti-inflammatory analgesic
Fludara		Leukaemia
Fungilin	Ambisome	Fungal infections
Gabitril		Epilepsy
Gonal F	Follistim	Fertility therapy
Haldol		Antipsychotic
Hivid		Antiviral HIV
Infergen		Antiviral HIV
Invirase	Fortivase	Antiviral HIV
Kaletra		Antiviral HIV
Ketrax	Ergamisol	Worms
Lamictal		Epilepsy
Leukine		Leukaemia
Limbitrol		Antidepressant

Lithium	Esxalith	Antidepressant/for manic depressive
Lodin		Analgesic and anti-inflammatory
Lodosyn		Parkinson's disease
Loprox		Anti-fungal
Loxapak	Loxitane	Sedative
Lusma	Theo-Dur	Asthma
Lustral	Zoloft	Antidepressant
Macrobid		Antibacterial – urinary tract
Meridia		For weight loss
Metadate		Attention Deficit Disorder
Mobic		Anti-inflammatory and analgesic
Naramig	Amerge	Migraine
Neotigason	Neotigason	Psoriasis
Neurontin		Epilepsy
Novantro		Multiple sclerosis
Optimax	Surmontil	Antidepressant
Orelox	Vantin	Antibacterial
Orudis		Analgesic anti-inflammatory
Pariet	Aciphex	Gastric ulcers
Pilogel	Salagen	Dry mouth and salivary glands
Plaquenil		Malaria and Anti-Lupus
Ponstan	Ponstel	Analgesic and anti-inflammatory
Prozac		Antidepressant
Requip		Parkinson's disease
Rescriptor		Antiviral HIV
Retalin	Concerta	Attention Deficit Disorder
Risperdal		Sedative in psychotic management
Ritalin		Attention Deficit Disorder
Rivotril	Klonopin	Epilepsy
Selsuh		Seborrhaeic dermatitis and dandruff
Seroxat	Paxil	Antidepressant
Sonata		Insomnia
Sporanox		Antifungal
Sustiva		Antiviral HIV
Synarel		Endometriosis
Tegretol	Carbatrol	Epilepsy
Tidomet	Sinemet	Parkinson's disease

Topamax		Epilepsy
Trileptal		Epilepsy
Trizivir		Antiviral HIV
Ucine	Azulfidine	Colitis
Vaniqa		Reduction of facial hair
Viador		Prostate Cancer
Videx		Antiviral HIV
Vioxx		Pain killer – analgesic
Vistide		Antiviral HIV
Volterol	Voltaren	Anti-inflammatory and analgesic
Zanaflex		Muscle relaxant
Zantac		Duodenal ulcer
Zonegran		Epilepsy
Zoton	Prevalid	Duodenal ulcer
Zovirax		Antiviral – anti-herpes
Zyban	Wellbutrin	Antidepressant

I must reiterate that many of these drugs have to be taken and many may have only a slight effect on hair fall – and certainly don't effect everyone in the same way, if at all. The list is long because of reports received over a long period of time, and they may not be mentioned in the literature that accompanies the drug. Therefore they should be remembered as a possible cause. You may notice that many, if not all HIV drugs, carcinoma, leukaemia, epileptic and Parkinson's disease drugs, along with many painkillers (anti-inflammatory and analgesic) and antidepressants – even aspirin – may have an effect. This list, although important and informative, should not be taken as the sole cause of a problem, but as an additional possible factor. Remember, too, that large doses of vitamin A can result in hair fall.

17

Hair Nutrition

How many times have you heard that taking this or that vitamin or mineral is going to help your hair? So you do so, and of course they rarely help in the way you would like so you continue to have problems. However, the importance of your eating habits and the way it can effect your hair should not be underestimated. It is a factor so often overlooked and misunderstood. And it is so simple to put right. After all, we all must eat, so why not eat what you should instead of what you shouldn't? Of course, it's easy to eat junk food or comfort yourself with sugary, fatty, salty, gooey snacks, or even have complete meals with foods that have little nutritional value but just taste nice. Yet following a well balanced, sensible diet that's going to enhance your hair (and you at the same time) can still include all the tasty – even junkie-things – you like.

It would be impossible for me to count the times when a change in diet has had a beneficial effect on the hair problems of those who have sought my advice. An interesting point though – and it still surprises me when it happens, and it happens so often – is when I start to enquire about diet habits. 'Oh, my diet is wonderful. I eat all the healthy foods, no junk, lots of fruit, salads, vegetables, juices, water, take all the vitamins – and my hair is still getting thin – it can't possibly be that!' These are remarks I constantly hear.

Even before I start discussing what they eat, I know what they are going to say – and it often goes something like this: 'I have fruit for breakfast, sometimes a bowl of cereal with skimmed milk [of course], perhaps both occasionally. No tea or coffee because they are bad! For lunch I have a large salad with lettuce, spinach, tomatoes, cucumber and celery, with an oil and vinegar dressing, and a slice of wholemeal [what else] bread. For dessert I have an apple or banana. And for dinner I have another salad to start, pasta, with vegetable and fresh tomato sauce for my main course, and if I have a dessert it's fruit or sorbet. I have an occasional glass of wine – never eat cakes, chocolates, biscuits or candy, and rarely eat meat. What can be a better diet than that?' There are variations on this theme: sometimes they eat yoghurt, or have a sandwich of egg or tuna, or have a cup of tea or coffee (black) – no sugar. And so on. You may be saying to yourself whilst reading this: 'That's me. What's wrong with it?'

It may all sound healthy and nutritious – after all, salads, fruits and vegetables *are* healthy. However, they are not enough to feed your hair follicles adequately.

Hair consists of protein, so eating sufficient protein is vital to strong, healthy hair. It's not sufficient to have only fruit or cereal for breakfast, however healthy eating fruit and cereals may be. Add an egg or two or ham or bacon or fish such as the old-fashioned kipper, and you have a perfect breakfast. Breakfast, incidentally, is the most important meal for your hair (and for you, too). Your energy levels to your hair follicles are at their lowest first thing in the morning, and they need a boost.

The second most important meal for protein is lunch. There is no protein in a salad, but if you add 120–150g (4–5oz) of chicken, fish or meat to it, you then have a good hair lunch. If you are vegetarian (and more on this later), a tub of cottage cheese or a couple of eggs with the salad or fruit would be needed.

Dinner is the least important meal for your hair, and it is here that you could indulge yourself with whatever you fancy. Another point to remember in your healthy hair diet is to eat between meals if you don't eat for more than four hours. After this time the energy to your hair follicles gets depleted. Most people leave more than four hours between meals, particularly lunch to dinner, and start to feel a little peckish and rather lethargic around 5 p.m. – so do your hair follicles, but you can't feel that! The ideal snack is fruit, fresh or dried. Or raw vegetables. Or a slice of bread or wholemeal biscuit, just enough to boost your hair follicle's energy levels until your next meal.

VEGETARIANS

It seems that vegetarianism, particularly among young teenagers, is becoming more popular, and although many children are brought up vegetarian because their parents are, young adults are easily influenced by their vegetarian peers – or they may read that this or that celebrity is vegetarian and think it cool if they follow suit. There are many degrees of being a vegetarian, beginning with just not eating meat but still eating chicken, fish and eggs. Others don't eat meat or chicken, then the more 'serious' ones eat no animal or fish but perhaps eggs or only cheese. Finally, we have vegans, who eat nothing appertaining to animals, only vegetables and fruits.

Before continuing, I must say that I respect a person's choice if they do not want to eat meat or other animal protein. But the fact remains that vegetarianism affects the growth of hair. Not everybody's. Much depends on genetic predisposition. Some people have such good hair genes that no matter what they do, their hair doesn't seem to suffer. It's like teeth: many hardly ever go to a dentist, eat sweets all day but still have good teeth – it's a matter of luck. However, as a percentage, I see far more vegetarians with hair thinning problems than any other group

Many vegetarians realize that because of the way they eat, they need to take vitamin and mineral supplements. And in doing so they think everything is fine. It's often not, and indeed sometimes can cause hair loss, by taking too much vitamin A for example.

I have said before that hair is protein. Proteins consist of amino acids, some of which are 'essential' while others are 'non-essential'. The essential amino acids include Argimine, Histinide, Isoleucine, Leucine, L Lysine, Methionine, Phenylalamine, Threonine, Tryptophen and Valine. They are most plentiful in animal protein and more easily absorbed in this way. The problem with eating only vegetables is that you need to consume a huge quantity to absorb sufficient amino acids to produce required energy, particularly teenagers, whose requirements are often not fully met. Without enough protein intake, energy is less available for tissue synthesis – the production of cells for tissues such as the hair follicles – whose requirements are very high due to the rapidity of hair-cell reproduction.

Deficiencies of calcium, iron, zinc, vitamins D, B12 and B6 are also common, and it is important to take all of these in supplemental form if you remain vegetarian. Blood tests will tell you how much iron or zinc or B12 you need to take so that you don't overdose.

SUPPLEMENTS

The above are all necessary and are naturally available in a well balanced diet. However, the metabolism varies among individuals, and the vitamins and minerals you eat may not be fully absorbed. It is rare that I do not recommend supplements because of this, even with what may seem an adequate diet. Often, for example, I suggest taking proteins based on gelatine, which is a protein easily absorbed for hair follicle function. I have them made especially, along with other supplements containing essential vitamins and minerals. Unfortunately, gelatine-based proteins are unsuitable for vegetarians, as it is derived from cattle (and may consequently be inappropriate for those of the Jewish or Muslim faith).

It takes a long time for any supplements to have an effect. And it takes a long time, too, for any diet changes to become beneficial. If you did everything you ought to in the way of eating correctly and taking all the necessary supplements, it would take over two months for the hair follicles to begin to benefit. As hair grows only half an inch a month, it would take about six months before you would begin to notice any changes – a long time if your trouble has been going on for some years, which is often the case. The unfortunate fact is that many people read about changing their eating habits and taking all the right pills, but get fed up with it if they don't see results quickly – and stop.

I assure you that perseverance will pay off. That means patience – do it and you will see.

In my last two books I recommended a '7 Day Hair Vitality Diet'. However, because a seven-day diet, in a way, promises results at the end of it, when in fact much longer is necessary, I am instead giving nutrition guidelines. It's easier, more flexible and just as good in the long term. And again, I must reiterate the long term.

GOOD HAIR NUTRITION

Hopefully, the importance of diet has been sufficiently emphasized in the previous pages. Taking it a step further, you should realize that all the food you eat is eventually converted to simple compounds that the body is easily able to utilize, glucose being the one that supplies the energy for all cellular reproduction – including the cells in the hair follicles (I have mentioned previously how prolific the follicle cell reproduction is). The following is a basic guide with many choices, and although it does not include (what you may consider) the 'unhealthy' foods such as cakes, chocolates and ice cream, it shouldn't stop you from eating them – or whatever else may take your fancy. The crux, though, is to have the underlying nutritional goodies – but you may wish to check with your doctor first.

The Perfect Breakfast

Any fresh fruit (which does *not* include juices). Plus: One or a combination of: eggs, a normal serving of bacon or ham, kippers, smoked salmon (or any other fish or meat), minimum of 6oz (180g) low fat cottage cheese. Added optionals: cereals, yoghurt, bread, any jam or honey, juices, tea, coffee, sugar.

The Perfect Lunch

Mixed raw salad or grilled vegetables or soup. Followed by a minimum of 4.5oz (120g) of any meat, fish, eggs, poultry or 6oz of low fat cottage cheese, with any vegetables of choice, including potatoes. For desert: anything you like, preferably something with fruit.

The Perfect Dinner (?)

As this is the least important hair meal, you can indulge yourself with anything you fancy.

Daily Must Dos

Drink 1.5 litres of water.

Not too much salt or high fat content foods, although you *can* indulge yourself.

No black tea.

Why no black tea you may wonder? There is evidence that drinking tea without milk can sometimes increase the likelihood of anaemia. Not adding milk leaves the tannin in the tea free to bind iron to it, therefore reducing iron storage. Although nutrition alone can cause hair fall and hair thinning and is often a prime factor in other forms of hair loss, it is important to keep in mind, in even obvious cases of poor nutrition, that hair loss can be due to other factors. I discuss 'Differential Diagnosis' in Chapter 23, and in every one of the similar-looking receding hairlines, a good diet would aid faster results – particularly, of course, in the case of anaemia.

A well-balanced nutritional supplement containing essential vitamins and minerals is also recommended. You can eat bread (preferably wholemeal), butter or butter spreads, use any salad dressings and anything else that may take your fancy.

You will agree that it's not a difficult programme to follow. Deliberately so. It's high in protein, and although some carbohydrates are necessary, you can limit them according to your weight requirements. Similarly, cakes, ice creams and pastries are not banned either. It may also surprise you to know that alcohol isn't forbidden.

So, to reiterate, the liver's storage of glucose lasts for about four hours, and research indicates that the amount of energy available to non-essential tissue, such as hair follicles, diminishes after this time. Proteins are absorbed slowly, carbohydrates faster. Whatever you eat at breakfast or lunch should be supplemented by a snack of fruit, vegetables or bread, in that order, after four hours between meals. I can further assure you that you will feel better and your skin will also improve.

18

Hair Tests and Blood Tests

HAIR TESTS

Like so many things, it seems that fashions change for no apparent reason. One year it's one look, the following it may be completely different. It's similar with hair styles, but it goes beyond styling as far as hair is concerned. Theories also change, and so-called 'Hair Tests' are beginning to find a certain amount of acceptance again when I thought they had gone forever, never to return.

About twenty years ago there was huge trend towards hair tests because it seemed an exciting and new method. Hair clippings were sent away to a 'specialist' laboratory to have them analyzed for vitamins and minerals. It was thought that the results would give definitive information on the state of your health and your hair. The laboratory would send back a mind boggling list, via a computer analysis, showing all your deficiencies or excesses of minerals and vitamins, and on that basis recommend the necessary supplements to put you back on track to a healthier you – and healthier and better hair.

It all sounded extraordinarily magical, but I'm sorry to say it was hokum, and the press eventually exposed the method. Hair from the same person was sent to three different laboratories and three different results were received. It wasn't necessarily that the analysis was wrong, but because each batch of clippings were taken from different sites and were of various lengths, the trace elements deposited on the hair or absorbed into it had to be different. In addition, traces of shampoo, conditioner, styling products and pollution, which are inevitably present, changed the results of the readings.

This is a method no longer used by respected professionals in the 'hair world' as far as I'm aware, but it is often used by nutritionists to analyze a person's ills. Many people also go to nutritionists for hair advice, thinking that their hair problem could be related to their diet, which may often be the case. As a result, they are given rather absurd advice based on the received readings via the laboratory they send hair clippings to. They are then advised to take multiple supplements, most of which are irrelevant to their hair, to correct the perceived problem.

I am not criticizing all nutritionists – there are some good ones, particularly those with medical degrees. Dealing with hair, however, is more complicated than simply addressing nutrition, even though it may be a factor and even if the analysis was valid in the first place. I urge you to think carefully before embarking on these expensive (and certainly irrelevant) tests.

The only hair tests that mean anything are trichograms, which test the status of hair growth and what your hair is doing or how it is responding to a particular form of therapy. A trichogram is used in scientific research to measure the hair's status to give a reasonably accurate profile. It counts the number of hairs per square centimetre, their lengths cut or uncut and their phase of growth. There are two methods: the plucking technique, whereby a small area of the scalp has all the hairs plucked and measured microscopically; and the phototrichogram, whereby an area is shaved and photographed at regular intervals to determine growth factors via counting the hairs.

We know from the plucked hair trichogram that, on average, males have more hairs than females per square centimetre – 312 to 279, which works out at approximately 10 per cent more than females and means that men not only have more hairs on their head, but that each hair is thinner in texture. This result is quite surprising, as one would have assumed the opposite. By microscopically examining the hair and its root, we are able to see, at intervals, the differences in growth phases and the degree of diameter changes. This has shown us that the thinner the hair's diameter, the shorter it grows, which may partly account for the fact that Oriental women, who have the coarsest hair, can grow their hair longer than any other ethnic group. It has also shown that hairs less than 40 microns in diameter rarely grow longer than 80mm (3½ inches), as discussed in Chapters 8 and 22 on 'Hair Loss'. Another point illustrated is that the hairs at the back of the head, towards the base of the scalp, have a smaller diameter than the hairs at the front of the head. The problem with the plucked unit area trichogram, as it's called, is the trauma of the plucking, which needs to be done at regular intervals. Similarly, the phototrichogram, although less traumatic because the area of scalp is shaved rather than pulled out, still results in a temporarily bald area. Either of these methods may be used in the research of new drug effects by pharmaceutical companies, but they are not really necessary in everyday practice.

All these characteristics can be seen by an experienced eye without expensive trichograms or tests. The changes seen also give us an indication of metabolic disturbances, as previously discussed. However, although hair can be an early warning signal of internal body changes, it doesn't tell us the whole story. Blood tests are needed to verify the exact cause of hair volume changes, sometimes together with a sonogram (an ultrasonic scanning device that provides a two-dimensional image and can give an indication of an internal problem such as polycystic ovaries) and other procedures. Looking at the hair can reveal a great deal, but eventually other tests may be necessary. The most important being blood tests.

BLOOD TESTS

The amount of information these can give is often crucial in the treatment of falling, thinning hair. My consultants, as well as myself, have a number of 'blood profiles' that we recommend in relevant cases. The tests are administered by a doctor who sends the blood drawn to a laboratory for analysis according to the profile we recommend. Alternatively, we send the client direct to the laboratory for the profile. Within a week or so, the doctor's laboratory sends a copy of the results for our own analysis as to how they can effect the hair. A typical profile, and one we use most, looks at all iron levels, including ferritin (iron stores), red and white blood cells, zinc, vitamin B12, folic acid and thyroids. Sometimes we ask also for hormonal levels and full blood chemistries. The problem with hormone tests, i.e. oestrogens (female hormones) and androgens (male hormones), is that they may be within the normal reference range but still affect the hair. I have already discussed this to some extent in Chapter 8 on 'Hair Loss in Women'. So much depends on the susceptibility of the hair follicles. For example, androgens. You don't need to have excessive androgens to have the hair affected adversely. It is known that much female and male pattern thinning is 'androgen dependent', i.e. it depends on the presence of androgens. But arguably you can have a high level and they have no effect on somebody who doesn't have genetically susceptible hair follicles. On the other hand, normal or even low normal levels can effect those more genetically sensitive. Similarly, readings in the normal reference range of thyroid, iron, ferritin, B12, folic acid, etc. effect some people's hair follicles more than others.

Then there is the question of how to read blood test results. In many instances all the results may be in the normal reference range, and if you have asked your doctor to arrange the tests, he may well say that everything is normal – and don't worry! But you do (and should) worry, because your hair is thinning and there are normals and normals, so to speak. There can be low normal, mid-normal and high normal. The highs and the lows can certainly be a culprit. Ferritin, which I have so often mentioned, may have a reference range of, say, 10–130. The results show a reading of 20 and your doctor may say, 'There you are – it's normal.' However, for hair, it's not. Optimum ferritin for hair is about 70. Anything considerably less can be problematical. Haemoglobin, by which anaemia is measured, has a reference range of 11.5–16.5. A 'normal' reading of 11.5 or even 12 can also result in hair growth interference.

Thyroid is another example of how low or high normals can effect hair. The thyroid can be very complicated, and those with hypo (low) or hyper (high) who are on medication can fluctuate, and this often causes sporadic hair fall. I discuss some of these in Chapter 15 on 'Your Health and Your Hair'. I am reiterating this because of its importance, and to stress that you may need to point out to your doctor (which can be difficult) that 'normals' are not always what they seem.

Biochemistries are sometimes required. These measure various liver and kidney functions, proteins, cholesterol, triglycerides, potassium, sodium, etc., all of which can have an effect on hair.

Blood tests are best taken after a fast of twelve hours, ideally in the morning before 11 a.m., without having breakfast. Subsequent tests should be taken at approximately the same time and circumstances for accurate comparison as the hair condition improves, so that any supplements or medication can be adjusted.

19

Frustrations and Difficulties

TANGLES AND SNARLS

One of the most common frustrations is hair tangling. It can be a simple tangle, leading you to tug on your brush or comb in an attempt to remove it, or you may have a very serious tangle, which is often referred to as a 'snarl'. I suppose it's called a snarl because of the immense frustration it causes, and you really do curse and snarl at it. Sometimes it is impossible to get a comb or brush through it, and unless you handle it correctly, it can result in a 'rat's nest' – a ball of hair like a nest and as hard as a tennis ball. Such severe tangling is unusual, and it results from a combination of circumstances such as hair colouring, bleaching, perming, breaking and falling hair – and most of all inadequate care before, when and after shampooing. You will already have read how to shampoo your hair correctly and how important it is to remove tangles first. Tangles should be removed gently with a wide toothed saw-cut comb. Start at the ends, remove those tangles, then go a little farther up and so on until you can easily pass the comb through your hair from roots to ends. *Never* start at the roots and *never* use a brush to detangle, although a brush may be used gently when all the tangles are out.

The reason for tangles is that the hairs' cuticles interlock with each other. The hair cuticle should be smooth. When it is raised, which can occur with various hair chemical processes or shampoos or back combing, they more easily interlock with the surrounding hairs – a bit like Velcro. Occasionally, if the tangles are particularly bad – you may have been out in the wind or slept badly for example – a light-weight conditioner smoothed through your hair first can be very helpful. It doesn't matter how much you put on, as it's going to be washed out anyway. And of course use plenty of conditioner after shampooing.

Fine hair tangles more than coarse hair because there are more hairs to tangle – and chemically processed hair tangles more than virgin hair.

KNOTS

Although they appear to be tangles, which in a way they are, they are quite different. They occur when the hair literally goes into a knot (see photograph below), similar to one that you may tie. Untying one knot under a magnifier is one thing, but if there are

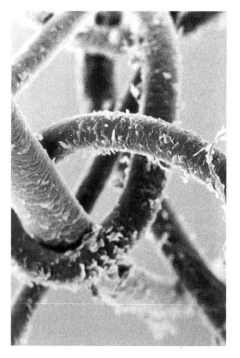

Knotted and dirty hair from wind

multiple knots, removing them results in the hair breaking off. Knots can be caused by strong winds on uncovered hair – more so in wavy or curly hair, and in tighter curls as in Black hair or frizzy Caucasian hair. This again emphasizes the importance of constantly removing tangles with a wide comb. Understandably, walking bare headed in a wind, on a boat, motor bike or open car gives a feeling of exhilaration, healthiness and well-being – but it's a bad idea. Ideally, you should wear some head covering – or if you really prefer the feeling of the wind through your hair, liberally apply a leave-in conditioner and try to comb your hair through during the course of the day.

SPLIT ENDS

Whatever you may read or hear, it is impossible to heal a split end. You can mask spilt ends with leave-in conditioners (which may temporarily glue them together), but as soon as you pass a comb or brush through your hair or shampoo it, they unglue. They can be very unsightly and cause more concern than is warranted for such an easy condition to cure. The cure? Cut them off. Ah, you may think, but I want to grow my hair long. Firstly, longer hair is more prone to splitting because of the 'weathering' effect on hair that has been there for longer, but split ends are not inevitable. Longer hair needs more care, as I have already discussed.

The biggest problem with split ends is that trimming the ends of your hair will not remove them all. Hair is of different lengths throughout your head due to the growth phases of each hair follicle. So you trim the ends about half an inch thinking the splits will be removed – which they will be – but the next layer of hair will be exposed with their split ends. To cut off all the split ends, you may think, must result in very short hair, which you don't want. However, there is a method that will keep the length. It's laborious and time-consuming – and you need a patient and friendly hairdresser or close friend to help. You separate small sections of your hair and twist it from the ends like a cork-screw. The various lengths will stick out along each section showing exactly where the split ends are and you just have them snipped off. It takes forever, but if you want to grow your hair long without split ends, it's very effective.

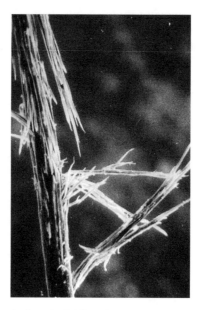

A close-up of split ends

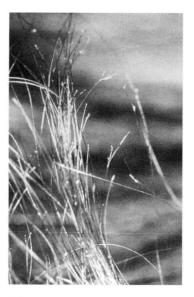

Split ends

FRIZZY HAIR

This often involves split ends as well, which makes the inherent frizziness seem worse. Frizzy hair can occur in all hair types, but most of all in curly, fine hair. It can be maddening. Frizzy is defined as tight, wispy curls, but in a broader sense it also refers to hair that has gone out of shape, sticking up in wisps and losing it's smoothness. Frizziness is also controlled by humidity and static electricity – and, furthermore, amongst the curlier hairs there are straighter ones. Hair is not uniform throughout, and together with variations in shape, there are variations in lengths, as explained in the section on 'Split Ends'. Making it even more maddening are the changes that occur during the day depending on where you are and the relative humidity. You can be at home, in an office, go out on an errand, go to a shop, take a walk, go into and out of air conditioning or central heating – all of which result in humidity changes and the degree of frizz your hair will have.

Hair expands and stretches and changes its protein bonds temporarily when wet or damp. During drying, the hair's shape is defined with whatever way you style it. You may dry it straight or wavy and it will keep this shape until it is wet or is being affected by humidity, when the hair will gradually revert into its natural configuration again. And this can change numerous times throughout the day. The way to protect from the 'frizzies' is to dry and style your hair with products that discourage moisture absorption into the hair shaft. Originally these products, in which the most active ingredients would be silicones (see Chapter 28 on 'Formulations and Ingredients'), were almost waterproof and were impossible to remove without multiple washes. Newer versions don't (or should not) do this. They are moisture resistant, lighter in texture, are effective anti-frizz products and wash out more easily. You need to choose carefully because some still leave the hair feeling greasy, coated, heavy, dull and even dry. I discuss what to look for in the section on silicones. Another point to remember is that little is best. Too much should be avoided because a lot of silicone used on wet hair to style it with the blow-dryer against frizzing up, can result in what I call 'silicone burn' – an unpleasant brittleness and dullness that is almost as maddening as the frizz.

LIMP HAIR

Many years ago I conducted a study of what was the most desirable aspect a person wanted for their hair. We randomly stopped 1000 women in department stores and asked them what they strived for. Over 70 per cent said 'more body'.

Limpness is really lack of body, whereby your hair doesn't feel full enough, its volume is less than you would like it to be, it lies flat, loses its style quickly, is too 'heavy' and is lustreless – each of which is depressing and demoralizing in its own way. The common denominator in all of these is 'fine hair', i.e. the diameter of each hair is thin. This is not to be confused with 'thin' hair. On the contrary, it's usual for fine-haired people to have more hairs per square centimetre because each hair takes up less space and there is room for more of them. In addition, each hair has its own supply of oil glands, so the more hairs, the more oil and less circumference for the oil to cover. The result? Even heavier and limper hair.

One way to add volume is to colour or perm, as these roughen and swell the hair shaft. Another is to use 'body building', 'volumizing' or 'thickening' products. Shampoos and conditioners, for example, can help. Leave-in products can also add volume by coating the hair very finely – giving the impression of more thickness. There are many of these to choose from, including gels, lotions, mousses and sprays. Again, as with silicones, don't use too much. Look on the label, too – Chapter 29 on 'Formulations and Ingredients' will tell you what to look for. You will need more of the bodying agents and less of the silicones – whatever you choose – and sometimes more than one product may be necessary. Use mostly on the roots because it is here that limpness originates.

A simple and helpful technique to further add body is to shampoo and condition your hair normally, apply a volumizer or any other styling aid of your choice and then begin to dry your hair. When damp, bend over and use the dryer with your hair hanging forward. Gently brush and comb your hair in this direction, following behind with the hairdryer. Pay particular attention to the roots, and when your hair is dry, style it in the normal way. You'll be amazed at how much extra bounce your hair will have – and bounce, of course, is the opposite to limpness.

DULL HAIR AND HOW TO SHINE IT

We have all had shiny hair at one time or another, even if only as children. Dull hair is synonymous with unhealthy hair as shine is to its health. Dullness usually goes with dryness, but wrong use of products can dull your hair, as can too much of a product, or you may allow your hair to get dirty so that the dust and grime forms a film and inhibits light reflection. Basically, the best way to banish dull hair is to have it clean. In addition, have it conditioned. Damaged hair doesn't shine as much as virgin hair because damage, whether it's from chemical processing or physical trauma such as rough treatment, raises the hair's cuticle. A conditioner used after shampooing helps to flatten the cuticle, and the combination of clean hair and smoother hair aids light reflection. It's the reflection of light that gives hair a shine.

It is a mistake to confuse dull hair with colourless hair. You can have an unattractive mousy shade of hair with wonderful shine, or you can have blond or red or auburn hair looking as dull as ditchwater. Many women I see have their dull hair coloured to give it more shine. It doesn't do so, although the extra conditioning that's applied after the colour is washed out will smooth the cuticle, and the combination of cleanliness and smoothness results in shininess – not the colour itself.

Another confusion is to expect all types of hair to shine in the same way. They don't – whatever you may try to do. The most shiny hair is straight, because straight surfaces reflect more light; the least shiny is frizzy and curly hair, whereby the light is deflected from the undulating surface in different directions. Wavy hair, provided the waves are uniform and smooth, can also be quite shiny.

There are 'shine' sprays or leave-in conditioners, which are mostly used on curly hair. They contain oils and silicones, which in themselves help to reflect light. However, to use enough of the product for this purpose means that the hair becomes very coated and attracts dust and dirt. The eventual covering of grime cancels out the shining effects the product may contain. Black women use these most of all unless they have had their hair chemically straightened. Straightened Black hair can be very shiny without a whole lot of gunk being applied. But it's not only Black hair that is very curly and frizzy – anyone with this type of hair should think seriously of having it permanently straightened, the reverse of perming it into curls.

Hair of uneven lengths or unruly hair where the ends stick out can look dull, even when clean and conditioned. Again, it's light reflection. Blow drying it correctly with a lightly conditioning styling aid will help to keep the ends flat. Or even a styler on dried hair applied with the palms of your hands will smooth down the misbehaving ends – and help to camouflage whatever split ends you have. So the dirtier, unrulier and curlier the hair, the duller it will look. And the cleaner, more controlled and straighter the hair is, the shinier it will be. It's really that easy. Forget about eating all the healthy foods to make your hair shinier – they won't. Surprised?

FLYAWAY HAIR (STATIC)

Another curious phenomenon of hair is its electrical properties, and flyway hair is simply caused by static electricity. How many times have you cursed under your breath at the way your hair sometimes seems to stick up all over the place – one hair seeming to reject the one next to it. You may even have experienced a mild 'sparking' when you have touched your hair, and you would certainly at one time or another have noticed that your hair is attracted to your comb or brush by rising to meet it like a magnet.

Another amazing property of hair is its insulation potential. Its electrical and insulation resistance is not far from that of asbestos (when it was used for this purpose). Hair is trybo-electric, i.e. it generates electricity by rubbing or friction. In this way it may accumulate electricity over a period of time and eventually flies away – one from another. The amount of charge the hair generates depends on the hair's cleanliness. If it is dirty or covered with sebum (oil secretion), the friction and therefore the triboelectric effects are reduced. Also, the moisture content has a bearing on tribo-electricity: the damper the hair or more moisture it contains, the lower the resistance and the less the flyaway. The drier weather and the higher you are – in the mountains for example – the higher the resistance and the 'crackling' greater.

The best way to reduce 'static' is to keep it clean and use a conditioner that clings to the hair shaft, so reducing friction between the hairs and therefore the build-up of electricity. Leave-in conditioners may well be best for this.

20

The Four Seasons

Seasonal changes in weather patterns, eating habits and metabolic factors often affect hair. I have already discussed nutrition and metabolism in other chapters, and the advice given doesn't necessarily need to be changed. It may, however, be obvious that summer diets are different to those of winter; our metabolism is also different. But the purpose of this chapter is to point out how weather factors can be overcome, along with social requirements of the seasons.

I will start with summer for no other reason than that perhaps it is the most enjoyable season.

SUMMER

Summer can be a perilous time for your hair. Those wonderful rays of sun that can tan your skin can blister it too. The same applies to your hair: the sun can lighten and streak it to a healthy-looking, sporty shade, but it can also frizz, frazzle and burn it if you're not careful. When combined with wind, heat, salt or chlorine, the results can be disastrous.

Many of you will think that because the sun's rays are natural, the change of colour in your hair that the sun gives is not damaging – but it is just as damaging as applying bleach. And, as with bleach, the effects are not just confined to colour changes. The sun weakens the hair's protein structure, de-moisturizes it and reduces elasticity so the hair breaks more easily.

Why your hair is not thought of when you apply sun protection to your skin is a mystery to me. Your hair is going to the same places, so why leave it out? 'Oh! My hair's dead anyway,' you may think (see Chapter 2, 'Is Your Hair Dead or Alive?').

The top layer of your skin is replaced in twenty-eight days. In this time your hair will grow only half an inch; if your hair is an average length of 9 inches, the ends will be one and a half years old and will have lived through at least one summer. The ends, therefore, will be bearing old scars, so to speak, so it is important not to make them worse. A hat is the best protection, but you may think them boring or unattractive or inconvenient.

There are simple ways to protect your hair from the sun without incurring too much expense. If you want to maintain your hairstyle, mix some high SPF oil-free suntan lotion with your regular hair-spray, half and half. Shampoo and condition normally and, whilst the hair is still wet, spray on the mixture, comb through for even distribution and style as usual. When dry, spray on some more. You will be nicely coiffed and your hair will be protected.

There is, of course, some effective sun protection hair sprays available, as well as some excellent sun protective leave-in conditioning styling aids.

For the pool or beach you will need extra protection. Chlorine and salt water can ravage your hair, so you should use a water-resistant application. There are many available, but your own mixture can be reasonably effective by shaking together some waterproof high-protection factor suntan *oil* with a thick conditioner. When thoroughly mixed, apply it along the hairs' length in sections, placing more on the ends; comb through for even distribution. The combination of oil and conditioner will protect your hair from chlorine or saltwater, maintain the hair's moisture levels and condition it, all at the same time. Re-apply after swimming. Since this preparation is greasy, it will give your hair a slicked-down look, which by the pool or beach is rather attractive. Don't forget that your scalp is vulnerable to sunburn, so make sure your parting is protected.

If the weather has been really unkind to your hair, a pre-shampoo deep conditioner should be used. But one should be used at least once a week throughout the summer anyway (see photograph showing split ends, p.110). There are many of these available to buy, but if you feel like it, you can make one yourself by whisking together:

2 eggs
2 half eggshells of olive or other light vegetable oil
½ ripe avocado
2oz (50ml) of purified water

Work the mixture in with your fingertips, leave for ten minutes and then wash off.

Guard against split ends by not over-brushing. Sun, heat, salt, chlorine and wind are enough to cope with; you don't want to have twice the number of ends as well. Hair tends not to do things in half measures, and if you are not careful, your ends could finish up like a shaving brush. Go gently and preferably use a blunt saw-cut comb.

Be careful not to pull the hair back too hard, and spread a little conditioner around the elasticized fabric to avoid it cutting into the hair. And, of course, daily shampooing and conditioning of your hair goes without saying – but that's easy in the summer.

AUTUMN

Even though you have tried to protect your hair during the summer, somehow the weather has really got to it. Now autumn is here, you realize that the sun, wind, pool, sea and beach that all felt so wonderful at the time have not been so wonderful for your hair. It has become dry, dull and split. This is all the more frustrating, as the more formal requirements of autumn mean sleeker, smoother and more cared-for looking hair.

The first step is to trim off the split ends – you'll be surprised at what a difference this can make. Secondly, remoisturize, as precious moisture will have been lost during the summer, affecting your hair's resilience, elasticity and shine.

You may think that rubbing in some hot oil will help. It won't, as you can finish up with lank, oily or maybe drier hair if it needs lots of shampoo to remove it. You wouldn't slather oil onto dry skin, you'd apply a moisturiser instead.

Your hair cortex, which forms the main bulk of your hair, is protected by the cuticle, a flat layer of overlapping cells. However, after a hectic summer the cells are no longer as flat or overlapping, and as a consequence the moisture in this vulnerable cortex could be considerably diminished. Misshapen, raised cells do not reflect light as well as flat ones, and dullness inevitably creeps in (see p.106 on

'Dull Hair'). There is little doubt that products such as deep conditioners for use prior to shampooing made specifically for this type of hair damage are better than home-made ones. They should be left on the hair for about fifteen minutes before shampooing out to give them time to pump moisture into the hair cells. You can sleep with them on occasionally, or if you're doing nothing social during the day, put some on in the morning and wash it off in the evening.

If you do want to try some home recipes, an acceptable autumn remoisturizer can be made with all manner of kitchen staples as long as it combines water, oil and emulsifiers. For example, mix:

2oz (60g) of soft margarine
1oz (30g) of butter
3oz (90g) of single cream
3oz (90g) of heavy conditioner

Whisk in a blender and apply the mixture to the hair in sections, working in well with the fingers. Leave on for fifteen minutes under a warm, damp towel or even overnight under a shower cap and towel. Rinse thoroughly and follow with your regular shampooing programme. A few of these treatments at frequent intervals will make quite a difference to the condition of your hair. When you are happier about your autumn look, an occasional application, say every two to three weeks, will maintain it. Look for moisturizing stylers and protectors, too.

WINTER

Don't let winter send your hair into hibernation. You can keep it alive and vibrant more easily than you think. The changes in temperature, humidity and the environment that occur in winter take their toll on you and your hair. Every time you step from a dry and heated home, office, store, cinema or theatre into the cold air and out of doors, your body and hair struggle to keep pace. Your hair alternates from dry and electric to floppy and limp. You may put on and take off a hat many times during the day, which ruins your hairstyle or look, as hats crush your hair and cause your scalp to sweat. It's not that I'm against the wearing of hats, but if your hair becomes damp under one and you then proceed to take it off when you go into a warm atmosphere, your hair will dry unevenly and probably have an attack of the 'frizzies'. Furthermore, heavy winter clothes can also make you and your scalp sweat, particularly on those cold, drizzly winter days. If your hair has already dried into an odd shape and then gets damp again, you are liable to end up looking bedraggled. By the end of the day your hair's a mess and you're very unhappy with it and yourself.

If that isn't bad enough, winter is the worst time for flaky and itchy scalps. Stress levels are higher during winter, and stress encourages the production of flakes and oiliness. Dissatisfaction with your hair increases this stress, and by midwinter you really have the blues. But this can be avoided, even though winter is the most difficult season of all for hair. The most important point is to continue daily shampooing and conditioning, something that is often neglected for fear of catching cold. However, there is no more danger of catching cold with damp hair than dry hair; it is simply that our resistance is lower in winter – wet hair has nothing to do with it. Less frequent washing also encourages a flaky scalp and lank hair.

Perk up your scalp with a tonic. To make one yourself (if you don't want to buy one) shake together equal quantities of witch hazel and mouthwash – 2oz (60g) of each will be sufficient. Add ½oz (15ml) of vodka and shake again. Apply the liquid to your scalp by parting the hair and sprinkling it on or by using a ball of cotton wool. Massage your scalp for five minutes and follow up with your usual shampooing programme. Your scalp will feel refreshed and your hair will benefit, despite the winter weather.

Diet is also important, but somehow the salads and fruit of summer don't seem so appealing when it's cold and dreary, and therefore people tend to eat more stodgily in winter and drink much less water. By all means eat hot stews, but make sure they contain lots of vegetables. If you can't face cold salads, eat hot cabbage (dark green and red), blanched broccoli, cauliflower, spinach and any other coloured vegetables you like. Also eat plenty of fruit – tangerines and clementines are wonderful winter fruits.

Even though it may be cold, try to get some exercise. Go for an invigorating walk for some fresh air, leaving your hair to the elements. When you get home, give your hair and scalp a treat by applying the scalp tonic, putting some conditioner on your hair, lying in the bath for a while, then luxuriously washing your hair with your favourite products. It will cheer you and your hair up so much that in no time at all you'll remember that, 'The hounds of spring are on winter's traces!'

SPRING

You can't quite put your finger on it, but somehow or other your hair seems to have lost its vitality. Whatever you have been doing to your hair during the winter, the chances are that everything spring stands for, in terms of renewal, regrowth and revival, has given you the resolve to look at your hair anew. You will want to resurrect it in some way by changing its style or colour; you may even want to perm it or cut it off.

What better time is there than spring to give your hair a vital boost? Firstly, get your style right. Styling and vitality are not necessarily complementary, but if a certain style and colour pleases you, then your morale is likewise boosted. Remember that if your hair is dull, colouring does *not* give it shine, it only gives it colour. Your hair will seem to lack body, too – one reason being that you may have grown it longer during the winter months. If there is ever a time to restyle and trim your hair, spring is probably the best.

The signs of regaining lost vitality in your hair are adding shine and body. I have already discussed this in Chapter 19 on 'Frustrations and Difficulties'. However, there are other things – starting with your scalp. The chances are that there will be some flakiness, so apply some of the home-made tonic described in the winter section previously, but in this case just mix together equal quantities of mouthwash and witch hazel and apply *after* shampooing and leave it on.

When taken internally, zinc can help cell reproduction. Used externally it can also be beneficial. Buy some zinc oxide cream (making sure it is a cream oil in water emulsion and not ointment, as this is not water soluble) from your pharmacy, mix it with an equal quantity of mouthwash and two large sprigs of crushed fresh mint until it is quite runny. Apply the mixture to your scalp in 1-inch (2½cm) partings and massage it gently for five minutes. Wrap your head in cling film and warm, wet towels for fifteen minutes, changing the towel as it cools. Wash out with your favourite shampoo and conditioner, and style as usual.

If your hair is particularly dry and lacklustre, apply a heavy moisturizing conditioner (after massaging with the zinc cream). Spread this all over your hair and then wrap it up for fifteen minutes. Rinse with plenty of warm water before applying your shampoo. Wash thoroughly, use your regular conditioner and style as usual. It may sound time-consuming – it is – but these two applications used twice a week for a few weeks will give your hair an incredible boost, new life and springiness (no pun intended). Spring does give us all an extra springiness – why not make sure it also applies to your hair.

21

Women's Hair into Older Age

The concept of how old is old has been changing, and whereas in our grandparents' day they may have considered themselves old at fifty, these days fifty (except to teenagers) is still young.

I see more and more women in their fifties, sixties, seventies, even eighties and nineties who want to take every step possible to maintain their hair. My mother, who died just four months short of her 100th birthday, insisted on me looking at her hair and supplying her with preparations well into her nineties.

And why not? The way your hair looks affects your morale at any age. The previous sections on PCOS, oral contraceptives, pregnancy, HRT and their hair effects can all be counteracted. With age it becomes more difficult but certainly not impossible.

There are many things we can do as we get older to keep looking and feeling younger. We exercise, eat healthily, use skin moisturizers, colour our hair – and as it loses 'body', have perms and use more bodyfying products. It is unfortunately inevitable that our hair gradually loses body. Very slowly, similar to our skin changes and muscle tone, the hairs' diameters diminish. This does not mean that we have less hairs in number, just that each hair gradually begins to take up less space – thumb hairs, for example, become finger hairs – 100 thumbs take up more space, look and feel more than 100 fingers (see Chapter 7 on 'The Rules of Hair Growth').

The degree of these changes depends partly on genetics but also on hormones – oestrogen production is less. All change with ageing, and none of us have the skin or body at sixty-five that we had at twenty-five. And just as we take extra care of our skin as we get older, we need to take extra care of our hair. And whatever your age, your hair can still look wonderful – if you do the right things.

The most important of these is frequent shampooing and conditioning – hair looks its best when freshly washed, and the scalp gets exercise as it is being washed. Daily is best, but if this is not possible, as frequently as you can manage – at least twice a week, though.

Each morning knead your scalp for half a minute: place your spread fingertips and thumbs over your scalp and gently move the scalp over the skull. Massage such as this should not be underestimated. Once a week or twice a month apply a scalp masque and a hair masque. Many are available in good pharmacies or salons. These should be massaged into the scalp and hair for about ten minutes prior to shampooing. If you want to make your own combined scalp and hair mask, whip together:

2 eggs
2 half eggshells full of witch hazel
Half an eggshell of vodka

Apply the mixture liberally to the scalp and all through the hairs' length. Massage gently and thoroughly for ten minutes and wash off with your regular shampoo and conditioner. Although this is quite effective, specific separate scalp and hair masks may give an even better result.

By all means colour or perm whenever you wish. Each of these swells the hair shaft and makes it feel and look thicker – and neither will make the hair fall out or make it thin. They may make it a little dry, but this can easily be counteracted by conditioning. Don't stint on using styling aids to add to your hair's bulk and condition. The choice of body builders, hair controllers, smoothers, shiners and conditioners have never been better. Again, none of these will make your hair fall out, and the cosmetic effect they give will add to your hair's appearance and your morale. Don't forget to eat correctly and remember that your hair is protein, so some protein everyday, particularly at breakfast and lunch, is important (see Chapter 17 on 'Hair Nutrition'). Also, in older age the values of haemoglobin can be reduced, making the eating of red meat, for example, important as well.

The hair ageing factor, I repeat, is to a degree inevitable, but with care you can slow it down a lot and have your hair look better than you think.

22

Hair Loss in Men

It is an unfortunate fact of life that the majority of men will notice a decrease in the volume (thickness) of their hair as they age. In Caucasian males (the most prone to male pattern hair loss) a degree of hair loss probably occurs in 100 per cent. This can vary between a slightly receding hairline, a thinning crown, an overall reduction in apparent thickness, advanced receding from the forehead, very thin hair, and all the different stages through from being left with only a 'horseshoe' of hair going around the scalp from ear to ear, to baldness. The size of the horseshoe can also vary considerably, depending on genetic predisposition and the age at which thinning started.

Caucasians are the most effected. Black races less so, by probably about 50 per cent, and the extent of loss is also less. Asians are the least prone and don't often go bald. An odd fact is that American Indians rarely, if ever, do either.

Male pattern hair loss has been mentioned historically as far back as 4000 years ago. At the time of the Roman Empire men wore their hair forward (like Julius Caesar) to hide their receding and thinning hair lines. And throughout history there have been countless baldness 'cures'. The ancient Egyptians used snake oil extract, bird droppings and stinging nettles. Other bizarre remedies included blood from pregnant women and newborn babies, the menstrual flow of virgins, bat's ears, rat entrails, bear's grease, all sorts of plant mixtures and saps – and so it goes on. Although these days they are a little more sophisticated, so-called baldness cures don't work either – at least the ones available over the counter don't.

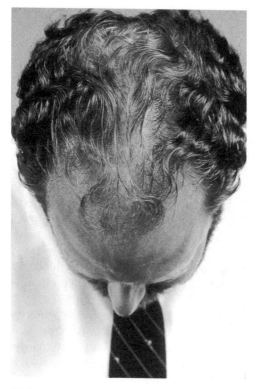

Male pattern hair loss

To start at the beginning, firstly, male pattern hair loss never starts before puberty. Perhaps in extreme cases where the genetic predisposition is strong, a small amount of hair thinning may occur pre-puberty.

There are a number of changes that take place coming up to, during and after puberty: the voice begins to change, becomes deeper and more resonant; sexual organs, testes and penis, enlarge and ejaculation becomes possible; the beard begins to become noticeable, the fluffier facial hairs get coarser leading to the necessity of shaving; hair begins to grow under the arms and the sexual parts, and hair can begin to grow on the chest and back. Every one of these changes is due to the increased production of androgens (male hormones), the most important of which is testosterone.

THE CONNECTION BETWEEN SCALP HAIR AND BODY HAIR

You may already be aware of it, but if not, look at the men on the beach or at a pool. The men with obviously thinning hair, and certainly those that are bald, have more hair on their body, particularly the chest and back, than the men with full heads of hair. An anomaly, you may think. It's not. Body hair and beard hair are stimulated and become longer and stronger by the action of androgens. Scalp hair, on the other hand, is quite the reverse when the genetic predisposition is such that the scalp hair follicles are more sensitive to circulating androgens.

It is odd, too, that bald men are thought to be more virile, but this is only because bald men are more hairy chested, and hairy bodies give the impression of extra masculinity. These have nothing to do with vitality. It is, of course, a myth perpetuated by balding men! Simply, it's all a matter of hair follicle sensitivity.

Asian men – Japanese and Chinese in particular – who are least prone to baldness also have least hair on their chest. Tell them they aren't as virile!

To reiterate then, male pattern hair loss depends upon two main factors: genetics and androgens (male hormones), which is why the medical name for it is androgenetic or androgenic alopecia – alopecia is hair loss and androgenic is androgens plus genetics. You can't have male pattern baldness without androgens; for example, there has never been a recorded case of baldness in eunuchs castrated before puberty. The proportion of androgens produced, testosterone being the main one, although playing a part in the degree of loss, does not need to be excessive. In fact, normal amounts of androgens or even sub-normal amounts can cause hair loss in genetically predisposed men. The more sensitive the hair follicles are to the presence of androgens, the greater the effect of the androgens on them.

GENETIC PREDISPOSITION

It is commonly thought that the gene or genes responsible for hair loss are passed through the mother's family. This is not necessarily true (see Chapter 27 on 'Hair Myths'): it can be from either side. Sometimes there is no discernable loss in any of the family, but a quirk or some predisposition from way back shows itself. However, whatever the origin, to develop male pattern hair loss you must have hair follicles that are androgen sensitive. You may think it's a case of chicken or egg – it's not really. Firstly comes the predisposition or 'sensitivity': without it, androgens won't effect the follicles.

WHAT HAPPENS

Androgens restrict the growth cycle of hair. By not allowing the hair to reach its optimum growth, which is approximately three and a half years and 21 inches long, it stops at, say, three years, then two and a half years, two years and so on. A shorter growth phase results in the hair being shed sooner – hair doesn't remain in the scalp unless it is growing. You may not always notice extra fall (although the chances are that you will), but a secondary change also occurs, i.e. the hair strands become finer, thinner in diameter. Two further things then occur. Firstly, thinner textured hairs resulting from hairs that were thicker also don't grow as long. Additionally, they take up less space, so there is more area between the hairs. Compare 100 thumbs (as hairs) and 100 fingers on the same site. The 'thumbs' would have appeared to be thicker, which they were, and stronger, which they also were, compared to the fingers that are there now, giving less volume overall. The 'fingers' are eventually replaced by little fingers ('pinkies'), lasting less time. And so it goes on until only fluffy hairs grow, or non-meaningful hairs as I call them – they don't mean anything to the look of your hair because you can't see them.

Research has shown that when a hair reaches a diameter of 40 microns, it rarely grows longer than 80mm (3½ inches). This appears to be a crucial stage, when often the hair loss can appear to accelerate noticeably. However, sometimes the deterioration seems to stop and the quantity remains similar for a long time.

There are numerous instances when the rate of hair fall doesn't noticeably change yet the hair is obviously getting thinner and receding. This is a slower progression and isn't noticed until it reaches an obvious stage, whereby the man thinks it has happened very fast and can't understand why he hadn't noticed more hair fall (see Chapter 2 on 'The Rules of Hair Growth').

Everyone loses hairs daily, even if you don't see them fall out, particularly if the hair is short. It's the replacement hairs that have become gradually finer; then suddenly there is an awareness to the loss of volume or the recession, again the thought being that it has happened quickly. The rate of shedding and change in diameters also fluctuate. Often for no discernable reason your hair seems to go into remission and remain the same for months or longer – or even appear to improve. However, the changes over a year or two are usually remorseless.

WHAT YOU CAN DO

There is no doubt that dietary factors enter into the equation, and a look at these by reading Chapter 17 on 'Hair Nutrition' will certainly help. But reading the chapter is obviously not enough: you have to do what it suggests! Particularly with adequate protein intake.

Keeping the scalp clean and exercised with daily washing and gentle kneading and massage – and not abusing your hair with hard brushing to pull it out – are also factors.

However, the primary consideration is to control the effect of the androgens on the 'target site': your hair follicles. There are two ways of doing this, either internally or externally.

Internal Treatments

The internal method tries to control the main culprit, which is di-hydro-testosterone (DHT). The testes produce testosterone. This on its own doesn't do the damage: it's when the conversion into DHT occurs that can be the problem. DHT can cause many of the miniaturizing changes in the hair shaft, and takes place in the presence of 5-alpha-reductase.

The latest drug to help counter this is Propecia (Finasteride). Finasteride was originally used to treat benign prostrate enlargement. It blocks the enzyme 5-alpha-reductase and helps to reduce the conversion rate and therefore the miniaturizing effect on the hair follicles.

Theoretically, all well and good. And it sounds a wonderful way to stop (and *they* claim reverse) male hair thinning. 'They' are Merck Sharpe & Dohme, a pharmaceutical company.

I met with some of their Research and Development and Sales people in 2001 after they had sent me details of clinical trials. The trials' results were as thick as a book and as intriguing as a good novel. The recommended dose to treat benign prostrate enlargement is 5mg a day. This dosage may reduce volume of ejaculation by 25 per cent, reduces the size of the prostrate by about 20 per cent and lowers

PSA (prostate specific antigen), the measurement of which indicates the degree of the prostate problem, by approximately 50 per cent.

At a dosage of 1mg a day for the treatment of male hair loss, none of these reductions occurred, although a small percentage noticed sexually adverse signs. It is interesting to note that in large long-term studies, 3.8 per cent of men taking Finasteride at 1mg a day noticed 'erectile dysfunction', but 2 per cent of those on placebo did, too! This indicates the psychological effects. In addition, the men on Finasteride noticed a considerable improvement in their hair after a year: 70 per cent reported no further hair loss and 37 per cent reported extra thickness. However, those on placebo also noticed an improvement, but less so: 44 per cent no further loss and 7 per cent extra hair. This was the front hair line and behind.

The crown area showed that 83 per cent on Propecia and 28 per cent on placebo had no further loss. Extra growth in the area was noticed in the Propecia users, and less so, but still significantly, in the placebo group. This also tends to indicate the 'mind over matter' aspect, but it does cast a certain amount of doubt on the methodology of the researchers. It's not possible for a placebo to help over such a long period of time.

Theoretically, Propecia should help. Yet there is a further problem: there are two types of 5-alpha-reductase – Type I and Type II. It helps to block Type II but not Type I. So men with Type I of the enzyme may be unlucky.

Because I also believe that Propecia could be helpful, I have instigated a study in my clinic along with Dr Jeremy Gilkes, a dermatologist. It has recently started and will continue for at least another year or so. It is too early to judge, but the results so far are not as good as those given by Merck.

As a form of treatment, I am certainly not against it, and those of you who wish to try it should do so – it may help and could help, but I don't think to the extent that it's claimed.

External Treatments

Minoxidil, also known as Regaine (Rogaine) was initially marketed as an orally taken drug for hypertension. It was noticed that one of its side effects was randomly spaced hair growth on the face and body and sometimes on the scalp. This effect arises from the drug's tendency to dilate the blood capillaries. On the basis of this, a 2 per cent solution was made and applied to the scalp. Studies indicated that this helped to reverse male pattern hair loss and the mixture was marketed, after FDA approval, about fifteen years ago. It has not lived up to its clinical trial results. The initial studies were based on hair counts (not dissimilar to Propecia). Observers counted at intervals the number of hairs on a circular area of scalp whilst using Minoxidil (and placebos). The method was brought into disrepute because it was found that the more experienced the observers became on counting the number of hairs, the more hairs they counted! Even the placebo controls had considerable increases.

Since then, Pharmacia Upjohn, the pharmaceutical company that produces Minoxidil, has made 3 per cent and 'extra strength' 5 per cent solutions available. Even with these, the results are disappointing. At first it seems they are helping – the solution darkens the vellus (fluffy) hairs and coats the hairs near the scalp with a stiffening film, giving the impression of more hair. All well and good – I'm all for improving the cosmetic appearance of quantity. The negative, though, is that the coating dulls the hair, gives it a brittle, dry look and feel, and often causes scalp flaking. Some of it is due to the inclusion of propylene glycol in the solution, which is necessary for the Minoxidil to dissolve.

I have not seen any noticeable improvement in the many hundreds of men and women that have been using it. However, intriguingly, even though they don't see an improvement, most want to continue using it because they think their hair may get worse if they stop. Perhaps a valid point and another example of mind over matter, since, theoretically, it would probably make no difference. Minoxidil doesn't effect androgens, 5-alpha-reductase or change the genetic aspects. Again, I'm not against its use. If you want to try it, do so. But be prepared, as with Propecia, for long-term use and not necessarily seeing the claimed benefits. However, there may be a possibility that the hair loss is slowed down.

Topical Anti-androgens

Taking an anti-androgen – that is, a drug that reduces or blocks testosterone and therefore di-hydro-testosterone or 5-alpha-reductase – can certainly be beneficial to your hair. The amount needed to have an effect, though, can cause side effects: tender breasts, loss of libido and lower sperm counts. And sometimes even large doses do not sufficiently reach the target of the hair follicle.

Applied topically in the correct vehicle – a solution that enables penetration to the hair follicle – they can be very effective. I have already discussed the use of anti-androgens in Chapter 8 on 'Hair Loss in Women'. With men, an externally dilute solution including cyproperone acetate (a very potent anti-androgen) and medroxy progesterone acetate has been found to have very good results. Recently, we included in the solution 3 per cent Minoxidil for some men. Not that the Minoxidil itself is beneficial, but it does help to dilate the blood capillaries, as explained when I was discussing Minoxidil. In this way the penetration of the anti-androgens can be more effective. Their use is long-term too, but there is no doubt about the therapeutic effect, whereby the hair loss is at least slowed, very often stopped and sometimes improved in overall thickness. Also, there are no side effects.

Many men want to try everything combined – Propecia, Minoxidil and topical anti-androgens – to cover all bases. This can also be good, not only because of their combined effect, but because it gives a feeling of satisfaction – almost euphoric – that they are doing everything possible.

Over-The-Counter Products

The number of over-the-counter and mail order baldness cures is extraordinary. You would think, if you believed them, that everything is so easy. I wish it were. There is *no* over-the-counter product that is going to grow your hair once it's gone. Minoxidil may slow it down, but even that in the long-term may be debatable.

I urge you not to waste your money pursuing the promised dreams from often spurious claimants. It is difficult enough with an ethical and knowledgeable professional, so don't believe the 'tests' and the 'results' of non-scientific, incorrectly perused and unsubstantiated claims – even if they say they have met all the criteria of proof. I assure you that they haven't. *Avoid them all.*

Hair Treatment Clinics

These should be viewed similarly unless they have an experienced, qualified professional in attendance – a Member of The Institute of Trichologists. If they ask for payment in advance, and this can run into thousands of pounds, leave! That is, if you're tempted to go in the first place. Unethical and 'cowboy' clinics are the bane of my life, and I have seen so many people taken for a ride that I can't emphasize strongly enough the necessity to avoid them.

23

Receding Hair Lines

Differential Diagnosis

During the course of only a day I can see as many as five types of receding hair lines, all looking similar but each having a different cause. And this doesn't include men – they are all women.

I have commented previously on how underestimated hair loss in women is. With receding hair lines, I claim there to be little difference in numbers between women and men, although the severity of the recession may be greater in men.

It is not acceptable that given a cursory look by their doctor, many women with front or temple receding hair are diagnosed as having male pattern hair loss. I find it extraordinary that this so often occurs when there is a completely different reason for the condition. Just because it looks like it, doesn't mean it is it. It's an easy way out for an overworked doctor who barely knows any hair physiology. Even the less worked private doctors sometimes fob off their patients with a similar diagnosis without attempting to find out more.

The term 'differential diagnosis' means just that. It is a diagnosis that differentiates one type from another and one cause from another. To find each cause is not necessarily difficult. It needs time, questioning, observation – sometimes blood testing – and often experience to tell one from the other. Take the four photographs for example. They all look similar. Yet the diagnosis for each is different.

1. Has been caused by anaemia
2. Is post-partum hair loss – the photograph being taken eighteen weeks after the woman's baby was born
3. Shows a pre-menopausal woman

4. Is traction alopecia – a self-inflicted hair loss caused by continual pulling

Although pictures 2 and 3 can be considered to be due to hormonal levels, they are not exactly the same, but similar in some aspects, and yet the recovery rates and results are wide apart. Treatment of each would also vary.

The anaemic woman and the one with traction alopecia in pictures 1 and 4 would also have variable recovery rates and different forms of treatment. The importance of correct diagnosis, therefore, is important.

All of the above have already been discussed in other chapters, and I also refer to differential diagnosis in Chapter 17 on 'Hair Nutrition' – whatever the diagnosis, nutrition should be investigated. The woman with anaemia, for example, was an obvious case of malnutrition. The others would also benefit by correct eating habits.

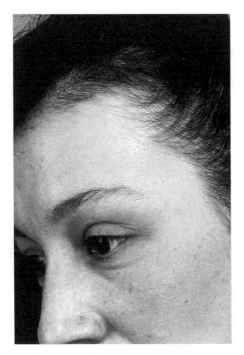

1. *Hair loss resulting from anaemia*

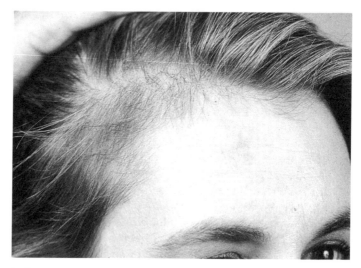

2. Post-partum hair loss

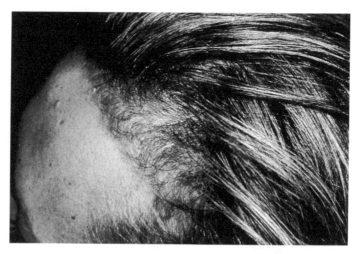

3. Pre-menopause hair loss

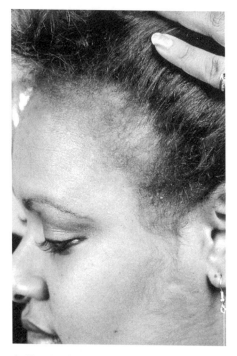

4. *Traction hair loss*

I mentioned five types of hair loss at the beginning of the chapter – these are four, the fifth is PCOS, as already discussed on pages 34–7.

The purpose of this chapter is to show once more how complicated hair can be – and not to necessarily accept a diagnosis of male or female pattern hair loss when your hair line begins to recede or thin.

24

Hair Twiddling
(and Trichotillomania)

In the 'Introduction' at the beginning of this book I mentioned that I have a weekly column in the 'Style' magazine of the *Sunday Times*. I have written on many aspects of hair and scalp and I get a large response, particularly on my website. The size of the response varies according to the subject I am discussing. To my surprise, the largest response I have had is the piece I wrote on 'Hair Twiddling' – over 3600. I was not only surprised but quite shocked. I wrote about a young woman of twenty-seven who had come to see me because she had a small bald patch halfway between her right ear and the nape of her neck, and her hair had become patchily thinner. It was immediately obvious that it was trichotillomania – a self-inflicted hair loss.

At one time or another most women play with their hair – fingering and twirling it – particularly when watching TV, at the cinema or reading. It is a habit that appears mostly confined to women – men rarely do it, although I have seen cases. It's not necessarily because men's hair is shorter and more difficult to grip – it's a condition that, for mainly psychological reasons, is more prevalent in women. Women with short hair twist and twirl their hair between thumb and forefinger, too, although the longer the hair, the more the habit seems to prevail.

It is normally a benign and pleasant habit, but something triggers it to become serious, leading to trichotillomania. Not only is it more common in women, but it occurs mostly around puberty or menopause. This young woman had been twirling her hair for about twelve years, starting after puberty. The first case I ever saw

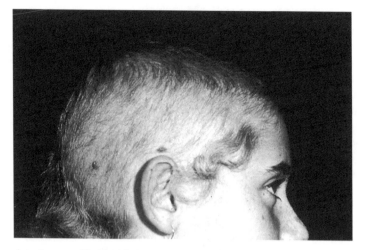

A twelve-year-old girl with a very severe case of trichotillomania

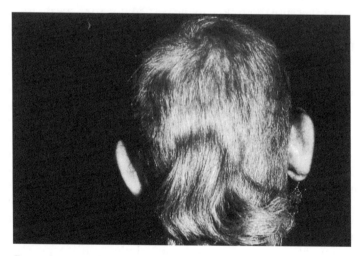

Regrowth as a result of treatment for trichotillomania

was a forty-eight-year-old woman (menopausal) many years ago, not long after I started in practice.

Trichotillomania, a definite self-inflicted hair loss, occurs when the twiddling gradually reaches the pulling stage, whereby the hairs are repeatedly pulled out one by one, eventually causing a thin or bald patch that can cover quite large areas. It's the hairs which cause momentary pain when pulled that are fully pulled out – so they test each hair first by pulling to see which one might hurt most, then tug it out. The satisfaction of this encourages them to pull out another one, and so on. It can go on for years because the hair from the pulled follicle grows back – at least at first. It's interesting, though, that the pulling takes place in areas which can be more easily camouflaged and covered with the hair that is left. However, there have been cases where almost all the hair has been pulled out, only leaving a fringe around the head – almost like a halo. Furthermore, women with thicker, more luxuriant hair seem to be more prone.

There are deep psychological and sexual undertones in this condition: from mild masochism, sexual gratification and attention seeking (because those close to the perpetrator, so to speak, are usually aware of the hair loss, don't know why it's happening, are sympathetic, worry about them and pay them more attention).

The sufferer becomes more and more perturbed about the loss of hair, knowing that they are solely responsible but unable to find a way to break the habit. However, they rarely admit to it and it needs delicate negotiation to let them know that you as a professional know the truth.

It's a difficult habit to break. Occasionally, psychological therapy is needed. There are other ways that require a lot of time and patience, too. One way is to wear thick gloves during temptation times, particularly at night (when the condition may be at its peak of temptation), so that the hair cannot be gripped. Another is to cut it very short so that it is impossible to get hold of; or cover the hair with a slippery cream or oil; wear a scarf over the head; or a combination of two or more of these solutions. It's a matter of interrupting the habit. Sometimes, playing with worry beads takes the mind off playing with their hair.

The good news is that the hair can grow back. If it's been going on for a long time, less will do so – or the hair may grow back a different texture. Those of you who repeatedly pull out grey hairs may notice they eventually grow frizzier, for example.

It is thought that trichotillomania is uncommon – even rare – but I wonder whether it is as rare as is thought. After all, it is possible that many of the afflicted don't want to seek professional advice. They may like doing it so much that they don't want to stop. It's only after it reaches a very worrisome stage that they may feel they must seek help. The huge response to my article seems to indicate this.

The condition is often misdiagnosed and confused with alopecia areata, a hair loss occurring in patches, which can look similar. The reluctance to admit to their doctor that they are actually pulling their own hair out leads to misdiagnosis. It's a secret they want to keep to themselves, which is another underlying psychological aspect of the overall condition (see photographs and captions, p.131).

25

Other Forms of Hair Loss

Rare and Not As Rare

ALOPECIA AREATA

It seems that the term 'alopecia' strikes terror into people because they immediately think of the bald patches that occur in alopecia areata. The word alopecia simply means hair loss, but it is the words attached that denote the *type* of hair loss. I have already discussed many, but not yet alopecia areata. The areata part means 'in areas', in this case specific areas of baldness that occur randomly throughout the head. It can also affect the facial hair (beard) in men, and eyebrows, eyelashes and body hair in both sexes. The last is very rare and is called alopecia universalis (universal loss of hair).

There is no doubt that the first sign of a bald patch causes panic for the reason that it is well known that a patch can become larger, another patch can form, and yet another. Each patch can get larger, eventually coalesce with each other and result in a complete loss of hair on the head – alopecia totalis (total loss of scalp hair). I am not surprised at the panic-stricken faces I see: their fear is understandable. Fortunately, it is unwarranted.

It is thought that alopecia areata affects approximately 2 per cent of the population, and of those about 98 per cent recover. The more advanced cases perhaps less, but still a pretty good statistical average.

It can affect all ages and all ethnic groups, but the available data can be misleading because some patients in some countries, particularly those in developing countries, may not visit their doctor or hospital. The peak age, it seems, is between twenty and fifty – a rather long peak age, but another example of its unpredictability.

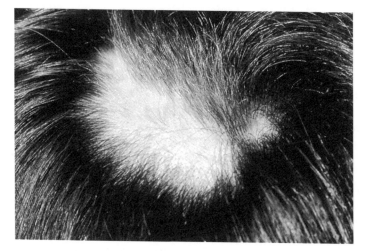

Alopecia Areata

The main diagnostic feature of alopecia areata is the presence of 'exclamation mark' hairs mostly near the margins of the patches. The number of these hairs depict the condition's activity: the more hairs there are, the more rapid its progress. Sometimes, there are no apparent exclamation mark hairs visible (although they may be there), but this condition may be diffuse (spread out over a large area) alopecia areata, which is even more rare.

They are called exclamation mark hairs because of their resemblance to an exclamation mark – thicker at the top and tapering to a thinner end, with the root a blob at the bottom.

The cause is not definitively known. However, it is nearly always associated with stress factors: sometimes triggered by a shock, an accident or a bereavement. There is often a genetic predisposition. On these points, I have personal experience: in my first marriage my first two children were girls, Susan and Helen, born two years and eight months apart. My son, David, was born two years later. The excitement of having a boy after two girls was immense, and David became the focus of attention. Poor Helen, it seemed, felt neglected, and at the age of two years and four months developed a patch of alopecia areata! I was dumbstruck. The patch didn't take long to cure – I made a mild stimulant tonic and applied it twice a day (which may or may not have helped), but we all lavished more attention on her and all the hair grew back. She has not had a relapse since and is now a grown woman. On the genetic side, my uncle (my mother's brother) had alopecia areata and so did his son, my cousin.

The condition also seems to be more prevalent in those that have hayfever, eczema and thyroid problems. It is also known as an auto-immune problem.

Treatment aims to stimulate the denuded areas with various substances, among them, very strong ones if the disease is long-standing. DNCB (Dinitrochlor Benzene) was often used, but its effect of acute inflammation and discomfort, together with other possible side effects, meant that it has become less popular. Cortisone and other steroids are used too, both topically and orally, the latter being rather frowned upon. Ultra-violet rays to get the scalp inflamed like sunburn has also had success. And a combination of all in really severe and resistant cases has been successful.

Saying all this should not distract from the absolute fact that the condition – miraculously – often clears up on its own with no help whatsoever!

FOLLICULITIS DECALVANS, PSEUDOPELADE AND OTHER CONDITIONS

I could have included follicultis decalvans and pseudopelade together with alopecia areata in Chapter 22 on 'Differential Diagnosis', the three conditions causing not dissimilar bald patches. But whereas alopecia areata nearly always regrows, these two don't. They are termed cicatrical alopecias, a hair loss due to scarring whereby the follicles are destroyed. Folliculitis decalvans is the more acute. Each follicle is attacked and it appears to be slightly inflamed, with the hair easily being pulled out. It seems that the nerve endings are also destroyed along with the follicle, so no pain is felt when the hair is pulled. The pulled hair root brings with it the follicle lining. It progresses slowly and is usually accompanied by a tenderness and even a crawling or tight sensation, which can sometimes feel sore. There are periods of remission when inexplicably it seems to stop – often not starting up again for months. It may remain dormant for a year or two in some instances. The areas of hair loss are definite, and unlike alopecia areata, the bald patch is slightly depressed due to the changes in the underlying tissues (the dermis).

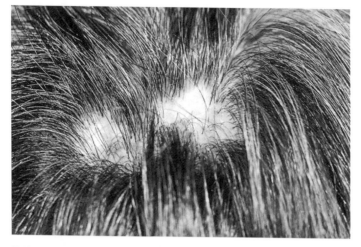

Folliculitis Decalvans

Pseudopelade can have a similar appearance, but it usually has smaller areas of loss. One dermatologist, many years ago, nicknamed it 'footprints in the snow' – multiple little indentations denuded of hair all over the scalp. There is no apparent inflammation, but as with folliculitis decalvans, there may be a sporadic soreness and inexplicable extra activity when the hair comes out more easily. It can also seem to be dormant for years.

The cause of either is unknown, but treatment with topical antibiotics do help. Systemic antibiotics are also given, but oddly don't seem to affect it as much as locally applied ones.

Lichen Planus and Lupus Eythematosis are two other extremely rare forms of hair loss; again, they are so rare that the possibility of you suffering from them hardly seems to warrant a mention. But they do exist, so I need to let you know. Each of these are extremely rare and you shouldn't worry about getting them. However, this book wouldn't be complete without including them.

26

Transplants and Other Options

TRANSPLANTS

I'm all for transplants. Done correctly, they can be very effective. Yet having them done correctly is not as easy as it sounds. In the transplant world there are also charlatans, and a good rule of thumb is to ignore those that splash large advertisements over the papers. Always choose a medical doctor, preferably a dermatologist or a cosmetic surgeon with transplant experience. Best of all, go to one that has been recommended by another respected professional and ask to see the results of other patients.

It may be difficult to grasp that transplants were first introduced in the 1930s and made acceptable in the late 1950s by Dr Norman Orentreich, a New York dermatologist. At that time the results weren't as cosmetically acceptable as now. Improvements have been gradual over the last forty years, more so in the past fifteen years, definitively so in the past five to ten years. At first, the results were often brush-like and looked similar to a Barbie doll's hair. A circular razor-like instrument was used to take out pellets of hair bearing scalp containing six to ten hairs.

However, to start at the beginning, the theory behind transplanted hairs and their follicles is that the recipient site, where the hairs are put after removal from the donor site, retains the characteristics of the donor area. We know that the sides and lower part of the head don't go bald even in the most advanced male pattern baldness (the genetic and androgen response in these follicles is much reduced or even non-existent). So by removing follicles from these areas and putting them elsewhere, they will still grow as they would have if they had remained where they were – even if they were transplanted to the tip of the nose! In effect, the transplanted hairs will continue to grow in the way they used to grow wherever they were put.

This is the basic principle and it all sounds easy. It's not. It needs an expert to do it and is extremely painstaking, needing immense care, patience and attention.

Hair grows at an angle from the scalp. The angle of growth is predominantly pointing away from the front and towards the back, which is the angle of the hair follicles. The expertise is to remove the donor grafts at this angle so that the papilla (growth point) at the base of the follicle is also removed. If it's not, the hair won't grow where it's put. Then, perhaps requiring even greater technique, the grafts are transplanted into the receiving area at the same angle. If, for example, they were transplanted at an opposite angle at the front, the hair would grow forward, away from the forehead, towards the eyes and be uncontrollable in styling. I have watched the procedure many times, and the two best exponents I have seen are Dr Walter Unger, based in Toronto and New York, and Dr Patricia Cahusac, based in Paris and London. There are others, of course, but I have seen countless numbers of results from these two in particular.

Whereas the first transplants were done in small clumps, similarly to plugs, nowadays the donor area is removed in a strip, and single or double follicles are cut off and inserted in small slits to where they are required. It gives an exceptionally natural look and the hair line that used to be a problem is hardly different to normal growth patterns. Another advantage is that the strip can give more access to more follicles, and there is a choice in the number of hairs that each follicle contains. Some follicles contain a single hair, some two, others may contain three and sometimes four. Also, the success rate is greater because very few hairs are wasted, unlike in the old method when perhaps 10–30 per cent of the transplanted hairs may have been lost.

Apart from treating the initial transplants with great care so that they are not pulled out with vigorous rubbing whilst shampooing, when they do start to grow properly, in ten to twelve weeks, they can be handled normally.

Scalp Reduction

When there is a large denuded area, a reduction of the bald area is often recommended prior to the transplant procedure. A strip of scalp is surgically removed, the size depending on the area that is to receive the transplants, sutured and allowed to heal – resulting in a smaller bald area and needing less hairs for transplantation. It sounds messy but it's not really. Again, expertise and experience is necessary.

The expert surgeon needs to bear in mind the probable progression of thinning in five to ten years' time. Although the transplanted hairs don't fall out, the thinning may have progressed and more transplants are needed. Therefore a good quantity of hairs have to be left for future use if necessary. Another fact to remember is that in a way you are robbing Peter to pay Paul, and Peter can't be left broke – meaning you can't take too many hairs, otherwise the back and sides of your head will be too thin to cover up. However, it is surprising how far you can go.

The new techniques are now also suitable for women who have thinned, and single or double transplants can fill in a thinned area or the temple region.

One final point, which to my knowledge only I have documented, is this: dandruff is usually worse at the edges of the scalp, including the back area. As the donor area retains all the characteristics when put elsewhere, it retains the greater tendency to flake off, too. I have seen, as no doubt many of those with this problem have, small areas of dandruff flakes on the skin that contains the transplanted hairs where there was none previously. It's just a point – nothing to worry about – easy to clear, but I thought you should know.

HAIR EXTENSIONS

The effect these can have on your hair's volume and thickness is considerable. They are an instant gratification for miserable looking hair, and an enormous styling and morale booster. Many women think extensions are God's gift to hair. At least they do at first. But it's not long before they begin to notice the drawbacks.

The old-fashioned hair extensions were put in by weaving threads which had hairs attached to them between the natural hair. They were weaved next to the scalp and tightly knotted at each end to secure them. Because of their proximity to the scalp, the thread, which had the hairs knotted onto it, rubbed on the scalp, caused irritation, consequently making it sore and sometimes breaking the skin. All very uncomfortable if left in for a while, which they often were. As the hair grew out, the attached weaved hairs would also become further away from the scalp, resulting in them having to be taken out and reweaved probably every four to six weeks.

This method is still used to some extent. But more often the hair swatches are glue-heated onto the natural hairs. They can still be uncomfortable and cause similar problems. However, the biggest potential problem is traction hair loss and breakage because of the pulling involved. Examples of this are seen in the tennis duo the Williams sisters, who have blonde or coloured hair extensions attached to the front hair, and the broken and receding hair is fairly obvious. Another drawback is shampooing: it is more difficult to do so and there is an extra risk of tangling the weaved hair into the natural hair, leading to poor scalp and hair hygiene, and flaky, itchy scalps.

Freshly done, it can look wonderful and completely change your appearance, particularly for special occasions. But it's not a good idea to leave them in for too long for all the reasons I have given.

Unfortunately, many women get carried away: they get used to longer, thicker hair and want to keep it, particularly those with fine, thin, limp or short hair. And they so often end up with progressively thinner hair due to traction and breakage, thus need more hair weaved to make up for it, making the natural hair eventually worse. And so it goes on. By the time they panic and finish up in my office, the hair can be in a really difficult state, requiring extensive help to improve it. By all means wear extensions, just bear these facts in mind.

WIGS

There's not a lot to say about these really, but they need to be included in 'Options'. A good wig can be almost undetected. It's the bad ones that give wearing a wig a poor reputation. The psychological effect of a wig can be enormous – even the bad ones give huge satisfaction to the wearers. The biggest drawback to wigs is the neglect of the scalp and hair underneath. Because a wig is worn, there is no reason not to take proper care with daily shampooing. The warmth under the wig gives a better medium for bacteria to flourish, making the incidence of flaky and itchy scalps more common.

There is an obvious and understandable reluctance to own up to wearing a wig, so much so that I knew a man who had a series of wigs with different lengths of hair which he changed every few days. Every few weeks he used to announce that he was going to have a haircut. He went off, removed the wig with the longest hair and replaced it with the one with the shortest hair to show his hair had been cut! Extreme? Not really. It is another example of the deep psychological significance of hair.

27

Hair Myths

The myths about hair are so numerous that they must rival those of ancient Greece. But whereas you know that the Greek myths are not really true, with hair myths you may not be quite so sure. Even now, hardly a single newspaper or magazine article on hair care is published that does not contain information based on one myth or another, and it can make life most confusing. So, once and for all, let's divide the myths from the truth.

THE OLD MYTHS

- *Cutting your hair makes it stronger/cutting your hair makes it grow faster*

  Neither is true. Your hair is not like a lawn or a rose bush where cutting can stimulate fresh growth. It is probable that this myth originated from shaving. A man shaves his beard off and within twelve hours his skin feels stubbly and hard – the more it's shaved, the more it seems to grow. The beard becomes stronger from puberty onwards due to hormone activity, but the assumption is that it has become stronger because it has been shaved so much. Another way of looking at this is to compare your hair to a bamboo cane: a long cane bends and flexes easily, whereas the same cane cut shorter feels hard, inflexible and stronger. In addition, cutting your hair short evens out the lengths, but your hair is not naturally all the same length and, moreover, the ends have less volume than the roots, so when it is cut short it appears to be thicker.

- *You can repair split ends*

  You can't. The only way to cure them is to cut them off. It is not possible to reset a broken-off hair in the same way as a broken bone! So-called 'split end-healers' may temporarily glue the ends together until the hair is washed or combed, but that is all they can do.

- *Hair gets used to the same shampoo*

  It doesn't. I think that this is a myth initiated by shampoo man- ufacturers to encourage people to change to their own brand. The same shampoo, used on the same hair under the same cir- cumstances, always gives the same result. Hair doesn't build up a resistance to a shampoo in the way that bacteria may build up a resistance to antibiotics. So why does it sometimes *seem* that a change of shampoo is beneficial? The reason is that your hair may have changed. You may have had it permed or coloured, cut it, grown it long or your state of health may be different. Also, it is like anything else that you're used to: a change gives you the opportunity to see things in a new way. But it may not necessar- ily be a change for the better. Once you revert to your old shampoo, this will likewise seem an improvement. Shampoo buyers are noted for their disloyalty, and manufacturers fre- quently take advantage of consumer dissatisfaction with other competitors. Very few of you are truly happy with your hair's performance so you try to improve it by switching products. I've lost count of the number of people who fly into my clinics from all over the world with the purpose of discovering which is the best shampoo for them. When I comment that it's a long way to come to find out, the answer I get is, 'You should see my bathroom!'

- *Frequent shampooing dries my hair*

  Quite the contrary. Shampooing, if done correctly and with the right products, actually remoisturizes. It is often thought that frequent shampooing 'dries out the natural oils'. Oil flow does not control the hair's dryness: it's the moisture level that does this. You can apply as much oil to your hair has you want, but without moisture it will still be dry. Oil is produced to keep your skin supple and to reduce moisture evaporation. Moreover, the oiliness cleansed away begins to replenish itself within twenty minutes. Anyway, who wants oily hair?

- *Frequent shampooing makes my hair oilier*

  You can't have it both ways, but people often think shampooing makes hair either drier or oilier. In fact, it does neither. 'The more I shampoo it, the oilier it becomes,' I have heard it said. You might as well say that the more you bathe, the dirtier you get. Clean hair shows grease faster than hair that is already oily; similarly, clean clothes show dirt immediately, whereas dirty clothes have to get much dirtier before it shows. Again, it is a matter of individual perception. Does shampooing stimulate oil glands? Does cleansing your oily skin make it oilier? Of course not!

- *Frequent shampooing makes my hair fall out more*

  It doesn't. Those of you worried about hair loss are often afraid to shampoo because of the amount of hair that you see coming out. However, everyone's hair falls out and all hair is eventually replaced. It may be falling out more due to metabolic reasons. Shampooing only loosens the hairs that have already become detached from the papilla at the hair follicle's base. Because you are scared to see how many hairs come out when you wash it, you leave shampooing for a few days, by which time you will get at least three times the amount of hair coming out. Don't be put off – shampooing your hair does not cause more of it to fall out. On the contrary, it may cause faster growth, as it has a stimulative effect on the hair.

- *Brushing your hair 100 strokes a day is good for it*

  It's not – it's bad for it. Brushing pulls your hair out, breaks it off and scratches the scalp. If you brushed your wool sweater repeatedly, you would wear a hole in it. Likewise, your hair can get worn out. A brush should be used as a styling aid only, not as exercise for the hair.

- *Tight hats cause baldness*

  They don't. If you wore a tourniquet twisted tightly round your head for hours on end, you would collapse before your hair fell out! This theory started because many men returning from wars had experienced some baldness and proceeded to blame it on the compulsory wearing of hats. The truth is that men go to war at an age when they are more prone to hair loss; it's just a coincidence that they wear hats. It is also possible that the stress of war or being in the armed forces can accelerate any tendency towards hair loss. Also, wearing hats usually starts at an age when the hair is more likely to thin anyway.

- *A cold rinse after shampooing closes the pores and adds shine to the hair*

It can also be very uncomfortable! Unless you are a masochist, I can't see the point of cold showers or rinses. They may be invigorating, especially if you dry yourself off afterwards with a rough towel, but they are really only enjoyable in retrospect. Do they close the pores? Not exactly. Cold rinses actually constrict the blood capillaries. The tiny blood vessels that carry nutrients and pick up waste products from the skin's surface need to be active for optimum effect; suddenly constricting them does no good at all to your hair. Does a cold shower create more shine? Absolutely not!

- *Grey hair is coarser*

If you have read Chapter 11 on 'Grey Hair', you will know that this is not true. Grey hair may be drier because hair goes grey at an age when the oil flow begins to be reduced, giving the impression of coarseness. Grey hair is also more likely to be finer in texture, as the ageing process starts to diminish the hair's diameter.

- *Hair can turn white overnight*

There have been many instances of this in literature and as hearsay, yet I have never seen a case first-hand nor know anyone that has seen it happen. Scientifically, it is an impossibility. The hair that you see on your head has its colour genetically formed. It can be changed only by applying a bleach or colouring agent. You can't go to bed with hair one colour and wake up with it another colour, or with a lack of colour in the case of white hair, unless you are Rip Van Winkle. It could happen if someone is in a coma for many years, where the colour is gradually lost as the person grows older. But overnight? Impossible! However, the myth must have started somewhere. My guess is that it is connected with alopecia areata, whereby clumps of hair fall out and are replaced initially with white hairs, but even this can't occur overnight. It is one of those dramatic statements used to convey the degree of stress somebody has undergone. Stress can affect hair colour gradually as the hair is growing, but certainly not overnight.

- *Pull out one grey hair and two will grow*

  How many of you wish this were true? What a way to make your hair thicker! What really happens is that you notice a grey hair, don't like it and therefore pull it out. The action of pulling out the hair can in turn rupture the hair follicle, and the replacement hair that will eventually grow takes longer to regenerate, by which time another, mostly grey, hair is beginning to grow next to it. When the hair that was originally pulled out does regrow, you have two grey hairs.

- *Baldness is inherited from the mother's family*

  It can be, but it can also be inherited from the father's side, or there may be no history of baldness on either side of the family and you are simply unlucky to have thinning hair. Alternatively, most members of your family maybe balding or have thin hair and you may have a wonderful crop! Somewhere in your genetic pool your genes help to control what your hair does. It takes two, a male and a female, to make a baby, and the genes of either sex can affect the onset of baldness. It is really just a matter of luck.

- *When a hair comes out with a white blob attached, the root is dead*

  Some of your hair falls out every day. When a follicle comes to the end of its growth phase (anagen), the hair becomes detached (the catagen stage) and falls out a few days later. The follicle rests (telegen phase) for about three months and automatically regenerates a new hair. You may notice that some of your fallen hairs have a small white lump at the root and therefore you think that the root of the hair has also been removed. However, this white bead is simply part of the hair follicle lining, which is similar to skin and, like your skin, is continuously being replaced. Furthermore, if your scalp is flaky, some of the flakes may also become attached to the hair. It is impossible for the root of the follicle to come out unless you injure your scalp tissue or have an extremely rare case of scarring alopecia.

- *Head lice are attracted to dirty hair*

  Dirty hair does not cause lice. If you do not wash your hair enough, there is a greater chance of lice multiplying faster, but they are just as likely to attach themselves to clean hair as to dirty hair, and can spread like wildfire in places where people play or work in close proximity, such as schools. When you neglect your personal cleanliness you are less likely to notice changes to your body and hair. Allowing your hair to become very dirty and itchy will conceal the extra itching caused by lice. When people do realize how infested they are, they blame the lice on the fact that their hair is dirty.

- *Dandruff results from a dry scalp*

  As I have already discussed (see Chapter 9 on 'Dandruff'), dandruff is more likely to be oily than dry. Your scalp produces oil (sebum) constantly. This is absorbed into the flakes, together with the serum that is often produced in flaky scalps. You see flakes and you think that they must be dry – how can they be oily? Well, usually they are, so don't slather oil onto your scalp to try to cure what you may perceive as dryness.

- *Dandruff is contagious*

  I discuss this in the dandruff chapter as well, but again, although we may consider that dandruff results from the presence of micro-organisms, all scalps are prone to it. The bacteria that cause dandruff are part of your normal skin flora, held in limbo, so to speak, by the resistance of the scalp's secretions to them. An over-abundance of these organisms can occur when the skin's resistance is lowered through other circumstances and the skin of the scalp is shed even faster than usual. You cannot catch dandruff, as you already have the makings of it. This does not mean to say that you shouldn't take care when using brushes and combs, because there are plenty of other things you can catch!

- *A lemon or vinegar rinse adds shine after shampooing*

  Nowadays this really doesn't apply. In the old days, before modern shampoos, you would have washed your hair with soap, either in bar or liquid form. The first detergent shampoos were referred to as 'soapless' because they were, and still are, chemically different to soap. The chemistry of these products is rather complicated, but the crucial difference is that soap is formed by neutralizing a fatty acid with an alkaline, leaving the resulting product alkaline. Water contains various degrees of hardness depending on how much calcium etc. is dissolved into it. The scaling found in kettles is an example of how water can harden. An alkaline soap takes the hardness out of the solution and deposits it on the hair as an alkaline film, dulling and raising the hair's cuticle. An acid rinse will neutralize this deposit, flattening the cuticle and adding shine. Lemon juice and vinegar are acids, so they act in a similar way. Modern shampoos, however, do not create an alkaline film, and neither do conditioners, so an acid rinse is unnecessary.

- *Don't use detergents to shampoo your hair*

  What are the alternatives? The word 'detergent' simply means 'cleansing agent' or 'having cleaning power'. Soap is a detergent, as are the solutions you use to wash your clothes, dishes and hair, although they are all chemically different. You wouldn't wash your hair with a laundry detergent, or your laundry with a shampoo detergent, but all of these are cleansers; each is simply manufactured for a specific purpose. There are, of course, stronger and weaker (or gentler) detergents, and various additives give them extra properties, but basically all shampoos *are* detergents because they cleanse – even my own products!

- *Colouring hair makes it fall out*

  There is no scientific evidence to support this – colouring does not make the hair fall more. It may sometimes appear so because colouring often starts as we age, which is the time when the hair may be beginning to thin anyway, so we blame the colouring when in fact it has nothing to do with it.

- *Women have more hair than men*

  Untrue. In a clinical study about twelve to fourteen years ago it was established that the average number of hairs per square centimetre was 279 on women and 312 on men. That's about a 10 per cent difference. It also indicates that men have finer hair than women. Because each hair takes up less space, there is room for more of them. Both may be surprising, but they're true.

- *Bald men are more virile*

  Not true. This myth may well have been instigated by bald men. However, it is a fact that bald men almost always have hairier bodies, particularly on the chest and back. The reverse is true with men with full heads of hair; the amount of hair on their bodies is much less, if any at all. Have a good look when next on a beach or by a pool. Hairy chests and backs are associated with virility, I suspect, because gorillas and apes have hairy bodies. It is thought of as being more male, just as lack of body hair on women is though of as being more feminine.

It just so happens that men with very little scalp hair have follicles that are more sensitive to androgens (male hormones), which makes it thin. Body hair is quite the opposite: androgens stimulate it to grow. However, it is basically genetic, occurring mostly in Caucasians. Chinese and Japanese men have relatively very little baldness and hardly any hair on their chest or back.

THE NEWER MYTHS

The above mentioned hair myths have been around for so many years that in an odd way many have almost become fact and difficult to dislodge, although, hopefully, I have to an extent dispelled them. The 'newer' myths are really more worrisome, as they have originated through heavy advertising, promotion and marketing by large cosmetic companies. Advertisers know that if you read or see something often enough, you begin to believe it, and it is in this way that the new myths have come about.

• *The Natural Myth*

This is really a psychological ploy adopted by advertisers. I wonder what 'natural' means. Products labelled 'botanic', 'organic' or 'herbal' also carry the connotation that they are 'natural' products. We could equally say that deadly nightshade, poison ivy, a bee sting and rabies are all 'natural'. Yet the word implies something that is healthier and better for you. On the other hand, 'chemical' has negative associations, although one way or another everything is chemical; the universe relies on chemical reactions for its survival. Water is natural, but it is composed of the chemical elements hydrogen and oxygen (H_2O). Plants are natural but their growth relies on the chemical reactions caused by sunlight and by soil composition. The whole of our metabolism is a series of chemical reactions: to digest our food we secrete stomach acids and alkalis, while 'natural' sunlight chemically changes the colour of our skin and hair.

Even when natural ingredients are used, they have to be extracted, leached, masticated and mixed with other chemicals to preserve them. Furthermore, natural ingredients all vary depending on sunshine, rain, wind and soil conditions. They can differ from year to year in exactly the same location, as found with wine vintages or olive oil, making quality control almost impossible.

Natural may perhaps mean non-synthetic (although this is also difficult to define). Synthesize is the opposite of analyze. To analyze you break something down into its component chemicals. To synthesize you build up a compound *from* its component chemicals. In the laboratory the quality of chemical ingredients is easier to maintain and so is that of the compounds that are made from them. (This is not to say that natural ingredients should not be used; I use some in my products.) But should the description 'natural' on a label influence your choice? The answer is an emphatic NO! By the time a natural ingredient has reached a commercial product, it is completely different to its original form. It may smell similar to the original and you may like the scent, so by all means use it. However, it is unlikely that an apple, avocado or orange cosmetic will be coloured by or contain the actual fruit, although it may smell like it. All it will have is the fragrance – which may have been synthesized. Truly natural expressed oils of flowers, herbs or fruits are many times more expensive. If you are buying a low-priced product, the chances are that the fragrance is not natural either. You may have read that the product you buy is 'naturally preserved' with no artificial ingredients. However, you can't preserve a product naturally unless you freeze it. Any plant, fruit or food will spoil without preservation, and the most effective preservatives are chemicals, which are found in all so-called natural products.

Hopefully I have made my point. If you are psychologically attuned to what is natural as a 'feel-good' factor, then that is fine. I am only trying to point out the anomalies: natural ingredients are also chemicals. A final word, though. The ingredients on labels are printed in descending order of percentages, the highest first and the lowest last – look and you will see where the 'natural' ingredients are!

- ## The Alcohol Myth

'Alcohol free' is another gimmick.

Most cosmetic manufacturers will have you believe that alcohol as an ingredient will do dreadful things to your skin, scalp and hair. Alcohol is thought to cause dryness, but this is not necessarily the case – it could be the reverse. There are many 'families' in organic chemistry, in which the family members have a similar basic chemistry. The way the atoms are arranged in the compound controls the individual characteristics of each member, determining its appearance and uses (much as in human beings). The alcohols are such a family. You have alcohol to rub on the skin, alcohol to drink, even a gas alcohol. There are also wax alcohols, oily alcohols and fat alcohols (called 'fatty' alcohols).

Some alcohols are drying agents, are used for that purpose and don't have harmful results. Other alcohols, such as the fatty alcohols, are emollient, protective, smooth to the touch and highly beneficial when dryness is the problem. In this category are cetyl alcohol and stearyl alcohol.   They are used extensively in cosmetics for this reason. An 'alcohol-free' product is not necessarily better than one containing alcohol – it may even be worse.

It may be of interest here to note that I can't ever remember seeing a bald alcoholic! I used to think that the easing of stress brought about by drinking was the reason for this, which may be partly true. What is nearer the truth is that alcohol can trigger a metabolic chemical reaction which releases the hormone SHGB (sex hormone binding globulin). SHGB binds more male hormones to it than female hormones, and therefore leaves less male hormones (androgens) to affect the hair follicle in male pattern hair loss. So alcoholics or very heavy drinkers may in the long term have thicker heads of hair. I am not advocating alcohol as a cure for baldness; it's just another way in which it may be beneficial. Cheers!

- ## *The Build-up and Product Overload Myth*

The terms 'build-up' and the newer one 'product overload' have led to the marketing of 'clarifying shampoo' – the term, I suppose, meaning to clear away any build-up or product overload, which are the same but have different terminology. However, they all seem to have become part of hair folklore. But I wonder what the marketers mean?

There is no doubt that part of the reason for the introduction of these words is the huge increase in the choice and use of styling aids together with leave-in conditioners. All leave-in products claim to add body or texture or shine or control or smoothness – or a combination, depending on what is required. To do any of these means coating the hair to a greater or lesser extent. This is how 'build-up' started, which led to 'product overload', which I presume means when more than one is used.

There are many factors, regardless of whether your hair is fine or coarse, straight or curly, coloured or permed, long or short, that contribute to the condition and appearance of your hair, so you may use a combination of products to achieve the desired style and effect. In other words, you build into your hair what you want it to do, look and feel. Or you could say that you build your hair to behave in the way that you want it to. So, in a sense, build-up is what you are actually striving for. But are build-up-removing products really necessary? The answer may be given by an analogy. In making up your face you use many products. At the end of the day you remove them with soap and water or perhaps a cleansing lotion. Hair and make-up products often have similar ingredients. You certainly wouldn't consider that your face suffers from build-up or product overload, so why should your hair be any different? It's not. You can remove whatever you put on your hair simply by shampooing it.

It's similar when you wash your clothes. Dirt, dust, oil, smudges, cooking ingredients and whatever else may build up on them. Then you wash them with washing powder to remove it all. Build-up is therefore just a term and not necessarily a myth; the myth is that it is dreadful and you need special products to remove it. You don't. The same goes for so-called product overload.

28

Hair Products

Cheap v Expensive

In spite of all that I have already said, you may still be wondering where to start. Choosing hair products can be difficult, frustrating and confusing. Where to choose them and how much you pay play a big part in this.

I often go into supermarkets, salons and department stores to keep me up to date with the extraordinary displays of hair products on offer. In one large pharmacy/drug store I counted 650 different bottles of hair care products. My local chemist, which is smallish, had over 130 bottles to choose from, not including hair colouring products, which have a display of their own in most places. Hair products occupy the most space in the beauty section, not surprisingly considering the billions of pounds per year spent on hair care.

The supermarkets offer the cheapest 'own label' brands. One supermarket had 250ml (8oz) bottles of shampoo and conditioner for 99p (I can't even buy a decent empty bottle and cap for that). I bought both to try at home. I also tested other brands. Of course, the shampoo cleansed and the conditioner conditioned. However, there are many degrees of performance, as there are multiple tactile, scent and colour characteristics in products. None of them came near to satisfying any of the criteria I would consider necessary, but it would be unfair to overly criticize products in this price range.

Mass market brands have huge savings in bulk buying. But the quality of raw ingredients varies: olive oil, for example, has finer or inferior qualities – so do cleansing agents, scents, colours and packaging. And very importantly, descriptively correct labelling seems unavailable in cheaper brands.

Prices are diverse and in most shops you are left to yourself to choose, needing a Ph.D. to understand the ingredient labels.

Hair salons, spas and department stores have an advantage here: a trained person can help. With hairdressing salons probably in pole position, they know hair and know how to use everything. They could have used the products on you when you had your hair done, too. However, this is not a true reflection of how they will work when you do it yourself. Your handling of your hair compared to that of a professional would be different and so would the end results. So don't expect a 'salon look' on an everyday basis. Personal attention also comes at a price, which is reflected in the cost of products.

Where there is not a trained person, most premium brands have more concise information on the labels and printed information available. Again at a price.

Good labelling should describe what *hair type* the product is for and what it is supposed to do, as I have already discussed

Designer brands when a celebrity hairdresser has a range bearing their name are thought to be superior. They're not – it is likely that they have all been made by the same contract manufacturer using similar formulations for other brands. The scent, colour and packaging may be different, but hairdressers, although wonderful artists, often know very little about the science of hair, chemistry of ingredient or formulation skills. The cosmetic chemist does this and has pet formulations. Most designer brands are similar in price and performance, and the psychology of using a famous-name product is not to be sneezed at. After all, if you think you're using the same as the celebrities, it makes you feel good (even though those celebrities also use other brands). The hairdresser is paid a royalty for the use of his name, which puts the cost up, but it is unlikely that they have been involved in formulation or that the product will perform better. Yet for the sake of an extra pound or two, you may well opt for the glamour.

Cheap v Expensive? Think of your face cosmetics: the better packaging, scent, luxury and feel of more expensive brands adds to the perceived results – and give an important psychological pampering and boosts your morale. They also look better in your bathroom. Hair products are similar: you pay your money and take your choice!

29

Formulations and Ingredients

A Complete Guide

In my last book this chapter was headed 'Understanding the Unintelligible'. Since then, labels have become even more mind boggling, and you need a Ph.D. to understand them.

Ingredient labelling is required by law, and so much the better. You should know what hair products contain, as you may be allergic to a particular ingredient or may want to avoid anything derived from animals, etc. The problem is that the list of ingredients in products is quite staggering – literally running into thousands – and identification is not made any easier by the fact that many of them have more than one name. I do not want to put you to sleep with a long scientific list, but unfortunately hair product ingredients *are* a long scientific list. The choice of products on the market is so enormous that it is not surprising there are so many ingredients used in their manufacture.

Many of the ingredients included in formulations are not necessarily intended to be beneficial to your hair. They are there simply to help the mixture to bind together, to stop the ingredients separating, to give it an attractive look or to act as preservatives. In such instances the ratio of the ingredient may be minute, but everything has to be included. All ingredient labels have to have the contents cited in order of percentages, with the highest listed first (water is often number one).

Many ingredients have multiple purposes: they may be humectant, anti-static and conditioning all in one, or they may be used just for one purpose, with another ingredient that does similar things but in a different way, or the percentages of what they may do vary – or they are better for some hair types.

The job of a formulator is extremely complicated and often requires a gift of foresight as to how the blending is going to look, feel, smell and behave – do what it's supposed to do. The look of the package is the first to hit the senses. The feel of the product when it is on your hands and on your hair is second, and then there's the smell. Their importance is not necessarily in that order, but dissatisfaction with any of them would either negate buying it in the first place or buying it again. Oddly, it's performance that seems to be last on the list – although it is the most important aspect.

Just to show some of the complications, the following alphabetical list contains the various categories of ingredients that may be required in a product. As I have said, many products straddle numerous categories – silicones being one. However, because of the importance of silicones, I have given them a special section, with which I will start.

SILICONES

If anything has had an impact on hair formulations and hair behaviour, it is the silicones. As a group they are rather unusual in an unglamourous way. They are not associated with plants or pretty organics, no nice oils are derived from them and their names can be frightening. Yet over half of all skin, hair and other cosmetics contain them. Considering they have been in existence for only about twenty years, their popularity in formulations is amazing. The reason is that when used correctly, they work! You have to be careful, as they were primarily used for their waterproof effects and as such were difficult to remove, often resulting in dry or heavy hair. The original silicones, dimethicone being one, were heavy, and dimethicone was originally used in the two-in-one shampoo/conditioner formulations, which proved unsuccessful in the long-term. They are now mixed and diluted with new and volatile silicones, making them significantly more useful. The modern silicones are the volatile ones (those that slowly evaporate), which can be excellent emollients, softeners and protectors.

The chances of you choosing a conditioning or styling product without silicones are almost negligible. The link between most of them is Methicone, but each has different characteristics.

The emollients include Dimethicone, Dimethiconol, Phenyl Dimethicone, Phenyl Trimethicone (gives shine), Phenylpropyl

Dimethicone and Cyclopentasiloxane-Dimethicone (often the basis for hair serums).

Volatile silicones include Cyclomethicone (most commonly used), Phenylpropyl Dimethicone and Cyclopentasilaxane.

Many have multiple properties and may be used in hair products of all descriptions – even in shampoos. However, their use in shampoos is a little questionable and should be kept to a minimum. Look at the shampoo label carefully and either do not choose them or make sure that the silicone is far down the ingredient list. Formulation skill is important depending on what results are required, and it should be remembered that less is best with stylers and conditioners, so don't use too much of your choice of product, and be even more sparing if two of the above silicones are in the top four ingredients.

Apart from the introduction of silicones into them, there are no really new styling products, just new names mostly, with a modification and jiggling of old ingredients to give specific effects. For your further information there are the following:

Laminates

These are basically used to give gloss and shine, the name, I suspect, being derived from laminated surfaces, which are smooth and shiny. They are a new name as a concept, but are really leave-in conditioners giving extra sheen. Their active ingredients are mostly silicones, often with multiple combinations of them. A small amount used on damp or dry hair spreads easily and, as mentioned, should not be overused, as too much will make the hair heavy and greasy looking. They are most effective in small amounts anyway.

Mud and Waxes

Their popularity may have peaked and they are mostly used by men for a greasy fixed and spiky style. Women may use them for a similar purpose. They are based on the old-fashioned pomades and are oily waxes (the old moustache wax used to twist long moustaches into shape was similar). However, now they have the addition of silicones with a variety of other ingredients, including polymers (compounds of high molecular weight), which are heavy thickening agents. They give the hair an odd dirty feel and greasy look. Fixatives include PVP (polyvinyl pyrrolidone) and names such as

Acrylamides, Acrylates, Butyle Esters, Karayagum and Copolymers. Their position on the ingredient labels, as with others, denotes their comparative percentage. The higher up on the list, the more fixative the product will be.

Greasers

These are thinner versions of muds and waxes, do not usually contain a polymer and are similar to the old brilliantines (greasy oils and creams). In other words, they are not really new products either – just a new name.

Other style helpers with newish names include glossers, shiners, smoothers, bodiers and curlers. In fact, something for everyone. Generally speaking, the smoother and glossier you want your hair, the more silicone you will need. The more 'body' you require, the less silicone and more polymer and fixative is necessary – so read the label.

OTHER CATEGORIES AND DESCRIPTIONS EXPLAINED

You may think it's a boring list, but don't let this stop you from reading it. Many things will surprise you, and the list will help you to understand how to read an ingredient label. If you think this list is endless, wait until you see the list of ingredients. I haven't counted them but it's over 2500! Most ingredients are listed, but there may be others introduced by the time you read it – things are changing all the time.

Compiling this chapter has required immense patience and research, and to my knowledge it has never been done before in a non-academic book. But for those of you with enquiring minds, the information could be interesting – it certainly was to me.

- *Antiseptics (includes disinfectants)*

  To a degree these are also anti-dandruff ingredients, as they inhibit the growth of, or destroy, micro-organisms on the skin.

- *Anti-oxidants*

  There are used to inhibit oxidation, which causes colour changes and rancidity in products.

- *Anti-statics*

  These reduce static on the hair by neutralizing electrical charges that the hair gathers from various environmental or product sources.

- *Botanicals*

  These are derived from plants through various chemical and physical processes. Their inclusion usually means that the manufacturer is trying to appeal to your 'green' leaning, although often the product will have extra preservatives – which almost defeats the purpose. There are a large number of botanicals but not that many are used in hair products. When they are, it is in very small quantities. However, some botanicals, such as witch hazel, capsicum, cloves, eucalyptus and other essential oils, can be beneficial in certain circumstances.

- *Buffers*

  These are used to maintain the pH balance (acidity or alkalinity) of the product and, although they do not necessarily affect the behaviour of the hair, they can affect the look of the product.

- *Carriers*

  Used as the base of a preparation; often called 'vehicles' because they may carry the active ingredients.

- *Chelates*

  It is often difficult to have 100 per cent pure ingredients. Traces of metallic impurities may be left over from the process of extraction, or absorbed from the environment or the container. A chelate forms a complex with these trace-metal impurities, binding them firmly to it.

- *Conditioners*

  This is a huge list, and the ingredients used depend both on what the conditioner is aiming to do (whether it is meant to be light, heavy, body building, remoisturizing, film-forming, detangling, etc.) and on the degree of strength required. The definition of a conditioner is something that improves the condition of the hair (or skin). This, however, is a very personal matter. Only you know what you want your hair to do, and you may achieve this only by trial and error. The description on the label, which should tell you what type of hair the product is for, is obviously a good guide. The ingredients in one conditioner may not be present in another, so you may finish up choosing the right product by a process of elimination.

- *Coupling Agents*

    These help to make ingredients more soluble and thus easier to mix or emulsify. Many ingredients are chemically or physically incompatible, but some manufacturers still combine them for specific reasons.

- *Denaturants*

    Used to make some alcohol-containing products unfit and unpleasant to drink.

- *Deodorants*

    Although rarely found in hair products, these are sometimes used to mask unpleasant odours.

- *Detergents*

    The mere name, somehow or other, has become synonymous with 'strong, drying, lethal-for-hair, should only be used for dishwashing or laundry'. Detergents, however, are defined as purifying or cleansing agents. They cleanse by emulsifying oils and suspending dirt particles, allowing them to be rinsed away. A detergent may be pure soap, shampoo or indeed a dishwashing or clothes-washing product. The choice is considerable and they are rarely, if ever, used alone. A shampoo would be formulated not only with detergent bases, but also with other additives to give specific effects. As with conditioners, the choice on the market is huge, and trial and error may be needed to arrive at your favourite. You can be guided to a great degree by what the label tells you (descriptions such as body building, remoisturizing, etc.), but some ingredients may suit you better than others.

- *Dispersants*

    These are often used to stabilize a suspension or dispersion of an ingredient that does not dissolve. They keep the ingredients separated but evenly mixed into the smallest possible parts throughout the preparation.

- *Emollients*

  Generally speaking, emollients are used mostly in skin care, to soften and smooth the skin. However, these ingredients are also found in hair-care products, particularly conditioners, and to some degree in hair-styling aids where the stiffening effect of some ingredients is buffered by the emollients. Products for frizzy, difficult-to-control, dry hair use them to help make the hair smoother, silicones, of course, in particular.

- *Emulsifiers*

  These promote the formation of oil-in-water or water-in-oil emulsions, which range from milky lotions to quite heavy creams. Oil and water do not mix, and an emulsifier therefore spreads them together uniformly throughout the mixture. They are what are termed 'surface active agents', i.e. they lower the surface tension of liquids, enabling them to mix together. In a way they are similar to detergents, which emulsify water and oil to enable oil and dirt to be rinsed away.

- *Film Formers*

  These are used mainly in styling aids – mousses, gels, sprays, serums and any other product meant to stay on your hair. Their purpose is to form a film after the solution they are in evaporates. The film can be hard, soft, malleable, shine-making, bodying or softening, depending upon what the product is intended to do.

- *Fixatives*

  These are not hair fixatives, but they do 'fix' or set fragrances and perfumes, retarding their evaporation and therefore giving products a long-lasting aroma.

- *Foaming Agents*

  Psychologically, a good lather or foam is essential for a shampoo. However, it does not necessarily add to the cleansing effect, as some excellent shampoos produce little lather. As long as there are enough bubbles to lift the dirt and enable it to be rinsed away, then the shampoo will have cleaned the hair. There are three types of foaming agents, and to some extent these subdivisions overlap. *Foam boosters* enhance the quantity and quality of lather; *foam stabilizers* decrease the tendency of the bubbles to disappear, and *foamers* simply produce foam – an emulsion of air in water. Foaming agents also encompass *detergents, emulsifiers* and *surfactants*. A surfactant lowers the surface tension between two or more substances, enabling them to be emulsified and to form a foam.

- *Gellants*

  Agents that form gels. They are used in many hair-styling aids, as well as for thickening purposes in other products.

- *Glossers*

  These give lustre, gloss or brightness and are used mainly in lipsticks. As with so many cosmetic ingredients, their use in hair products is becoming more common, particularly the silicone derivatives (methicones).

- *Humectants*

  Absorb water and hold and retain moisture. They are therefore used to prevent products drying out and to add moisture to skin and hair. Care should be taken when using humectants, as their moisture-absorbing properties may backfire and they may absorb moisture from the surface of the scalp. They are meant to moisturize, but their drawback in hair products is that they can give the hair a limp look and feel, as well as a peculiar dryness if used over a long period.

- *Lubricants*

  These reduce friction, smooth the hair and add shine. They can make the hair heavy, but in some circumstances can be beneficial, particularly for protection purposes.

- *Moisturizers*

  Increase the moisture content of the skin and hair, and add softness and control to frizzy hair. They can, however, be unsuitable for use on limp, thin hair.

- *Opacifiers*

  Used to make liquids and creams opaque so that they appear thicker or richer. Opacifiers do not add to the performance of the product.

- *Pearlants*

  Formally popular as a marketing gimmick in shampoos and conditioners, pearlants are now used for their supposed beneficial properties or to impart a richer, pearly texture.

- *Plasticizers*

  These make film-forming ingredients more flexible and softer. They are also used to denature alcohol (methyl), making it unfit to drink.

- *Preservatives*

  These are found in all cosmetics, including hair preparations. Each preservative controls the growth of specific micro-organisms that can cause spoilage. One preservative is often insufficient because different ingredients may grow different micro-organisms, and each ingredient may be affected in a different way. The shelf-life of a preparation is of immense importance and a lot of work goes into testing it. There are many proprietary preservatives that are a combination of several. The percentage of preservative in a product is very small, and you can see that they are near the bottom of the list of contents on the label.

- *Propellants*

  These are used to propel the product from its container, being mainly found in mousses and hair sprays.

- *Proteins*

  Proteins should really be eaten! However, they are also used in hair-care products, and when applied externally they coat the hair shaft, helping to strengthen it. Proteins are contained in many hair preparations in one form or another, and choosing the right one can be a triumph of formulation. There is absolutely no truth in the theory that because hair is nearly 100 per cent protein, proteins in hair products must be beneficial to its growth. Although there are naturally occurring complex combinations of amino acids of which proteins are composed, neither externally applied amino acids nor proteins are absorbed into the hair shaft or the hair root. They may help to strengthen hair, but only in their binding and coating capacity.

- *Refatting Agents*

  These help to add oily materials to the skin and hair. Remember, dryness of hair is due to loss of moisture, not loss of oil. Adding oiliness makes the hair heavy if it is fine and limp, and attracts dust and dirt. Refatting agents can, however, be occlusive, and are sometimes used in treatment masks for dry hair or skin to prevent temporary moisture evaporation.

- *Resins*

  There are many forms of resin and they are often a component of hair fixatives such as sprays, gels and mousses. They are either solid or semi-solid substances. Resins are often obtained from plants, but equally effective ones can be made synthetically. Various substances are used to dissolve the resin; when the solvent evaporates, a film of resin is left on the hair.

- *Solvents*

  In themselves, solvents are often beneficial. They are used to dissolve other substances to enable them to be used in the way the formulator wants them to. The most commonly used solvent is alcohol, which, in its liquid form of methyl or ethyl alcohol, can be drying, so oils and fats as well as fatty alcohols may be added to counteract this effect.

- *Stabilizers*

  These are usually additives with no beneficial effect except to stabilize an emulsion or suspension and to stop it separating.

- *Stimulants*

  Produce a temporary increase in the activity of other ingredients, but can also act as a stimulant in their own right. They are often used in scalp tonics, in small quantities, and give an invigorating, tingly feeling to the scalp.

- *Sunscreens*

  Their use in skin preparations is well known, but it is only fairly recently that they have been included in hair products – and why not! Hair is just as prone to sun damage as skin, but as it doesn't become inflamed or sore, by the time you have realized this, it is often too late. The biggest problem with sunscreens is that most are heavy and need to be spread evenly in a light coating. They can also attract dirt. Some people are sensitive to certain ones, so it is important to know which sunscreen(s) the product contains. UV-A absorbs the longer wavelengths and UV-B the shorter ones; many sunscreens absorb them both.

- *Surfactants (Surface-Active Agents)*

  You may be getting a little fed up by now with detergents, emulsifiers, foaming agents, foam boosters and stabilizers – they all seem to do a similar job. This is true to an extent. But surfactants also lower the surface tension between the many apparently incompatible materials found in soaps, detergents, wetting agents, foamers, solubilizers, emulsifiers, etc. Surfactants act as negatively charged (anionic), positively charged (cationic), non-ionic (neutral) and amphoteric (anionic *and* cationic) agents. This makes them suitable for many purposes, and they are included in a large range of products, not only as beneficial components to the hair, but for formulation purposes, too.

- *Suspending Agents*

  These are used to keep finely divided, solid particles suspended in a solution so that they don't separate. Although not found that often, they have been included just in case.

- *Thickeners*

  As their name suggests, these are used to give lotions and creams a thicker consistency. Many of them also fall into other categories and are used for other purposes.

- *Thixotropes*

  You have never heard of them? Although not often used, they do have an interesting property. Thixotropic gels or emulsions become more fluid and easier running when shaken or stirred, and their inclusion in a product enables quite thick substances to be expressed more easily from their containers.

- *Vegetable Oils*

  These speak for themselves. Olive oil, almond oil, sunflower oil, corn oil, walnut oil – the list is long.

- *Vitamins*

  Some products contain vitamins as a marketing gimmick. There is no evidence, in my experience, or any true scientific data to support the claims that they are absorbed into the hair. They may, however, be used to coat or smooth the hair shaft. Vitamins, like proteins, are best when eaten!

- *Waxes*

  These are used less than you might have thought. However, waxes are quite often required in small amounts in skin and hair cosmetics, although too much wax may make the preparation over-greasy or heavy. Some products, though, are called a 'wax', wanting that effect for styling.

- *Wetting Agents*

  These help in literally wetting the surfaces on which they are used. They are *surfactants* (surface active agents), and may in some circumstances give a softening effect.

All the above are included in the ingredient list to explain what they are for, and can be referred to by this key to ingredient letters.

KEY TO INGREDIENTS

Anti-dandruff AD	Emollients EL	Proteins PT
Anti-oxidants AO	Emulsifiers ES	Refatting Agents RA
Anti-septics AP	Film Formers FF	Resins RS
Anti-statics AS	Fixatives FX	Silicones SI
Astringents A	Foaming Agents FA	Solvents SO
Botanicals BO	Gellants GE	Stabilizers SB
Buffers BF	Glossers GL	Stimulants ST
Carriers CR	Humectants HU	Sunscreens SS
Chelates CH	Lubricants LU	Surfactants SF
Conditioners CO	Moisturizers MO	Suspending Agents SA
Coupling Agents CA	Opacifiers OP	Thickeners TK
Denaturants DN	Pearlants PE	Thixotropes TX
Deodorants DO	Plasticizers PL	Vegetable Oils VA
Detergents DT	Preservatives PR	Vitamins VT
Dispersants DS	Propellants PP	Waxes WX
		Wetting Agents WA

INGREDIENTS

1-Docosanol *EL TK*

1 Lysine lauryl methionine *AD*

2-Bromo–2-nitropropane–1,3-diol *AD AP PR*

2-Butyl octanol *EL*

2-Ethylhexyl hexamdecanoate *EL*

2-Ethylhexyl isostearate *EL SO*

2-Octyldodecyl alcohol *ES*

2-Octyldodecyl erucate *EL*

2-Octyldodecyl lactate *EL*

2-Octyldodecyl oleate *EL*

2-Octyldodecyl ricinoleate *EL*

2-Phenyl-benzimidazole-5-sulfonic acid *SS*

3-Benzylidene camphor *SS*

3-Methyl–1,3-butanediol *EL*

4-Isopropyl dibenzoyl methane *SS*

4-Methyl benzenesulfonamide *RS*

4-Methylbenzylidene camphor *SS*

5-Bromo–5-nitro–1,3-dioxane *PR*

7-Ethyl bicyclooxazolidine *PR*

Abietic acid *DO*

Acacia gum (Acacia ssp.) *BO*

Acetamide MEA *AS CO HU*

Acetamido propyl trimonium chloride *AS MO*

Aceyl tributyl citrate *PL*

Acetyl triethyl citrate *PL*

Acetylated glycol stearate *EL*

Acetylated hydrogenated lanolin *EL*

Acetylated hydrogenated lard glyceride *EL ES*

Acetylated hydrogenated vegetable glyceride *EL*

ES

Acetylated lanolin *EL FF*

Acetylated lanolin alcohol *EL*

Acetylated lard glyceride *EL*

Acetylated palm kernel glycerides *EL*

Acrylates C10-C30 alkyl acrylate crosspolymer *TK*

Acrylates copolymer *TK*

Acrylates-stearate–50 acrylate copolymer *TK*

Acrylates-VA crosspolymer *SB TK*

Acrylates / steareth–20 methacrylate copolymer *TK*

Acrylic acid / acrylonitrogens copolymer *ES GE TK*

Adenosine phosphate *HU*

Adenosine triphosphate *MO*

Agar *GE*

Agromony extract (Agrimonia eupatoria L.) *BO*

Albumen *PT*

Alcohol *PR*

Alfalfa extract *BO*

Algae extract *BO MO*

Algae extract (Fucus vesiculosus) *MO*

Algae extract (Laminaria spp.) *BO*

Algin *GE SA TK*

Alkyl dimethyl betaine *AS SF*

Alkylated polycincylpyrrolidone *FF*

Alkylated polyvinylpyrrolidone *DS*

Alkyldimethylamine oxide *FA SB SF*

Allantoin acetyl methionine *AD*

Allantoin glycyrrhetinic acid *AD*

Allantoin polygalacturonic acid *AD*

Aloe *BO MO*

Aloe vera extracts *BO MO*

Aloe vera gel, condensed *BO MO*

Aloe vera gel, decolorized *BO MO*

Aloe vera gel, food grade *BO MO*

Aloe vera gel freeze-dried powder *MO*

Alpine Veronica extract (Veronica alpina) *BO*

Althea extract (Althea officinalis) *BO*

Aluminium citrate *A*

Aluminium distearate *GE*

Aluminium lactate *A*

Aluminium magnesium hydroxystearate *EL TK*

Aluminium PCA *AP*

Aluminium salt octenyl succinate *LU*

Aluminium tristearate *GE*

Amino bispropyl dimethicone *SI*

Ammonium acrylates-acrylonitrogens copolymer *FF GE TK*

Ammonium alginate *TK*

Ammonium C12–15 alkyl sulfate *SF*

Ammonium cocoyl sarcosinate *SF*

Ammonium crylates acrylonitrogens copolymer *ES*

Ammonium iodide *AD*

Ammonium laureth sulfate *DT FA SF*

Ammonium laureth–5 sulfate *FA SF*

Ammonium laureth–12 sulfate *FA SF*

Ammonium lauroyl sarcosinate *SF*

Ammonium lauryl sulfate
  DT FA
Ammonium lauryl
  sulfosuccinate *FA SF*
Ammonium myreth sulfate
  FA SF
Ammonium nonoxynol 4
  sulfate *FA SF*
Amniotic fluid *MO*
Amodimethicone *LU SI*
AMP-isostearoyl
  hydrolyzed soy protein
  EL
AMPD isostearoyl
  hydrolyzed collagen *PL*
Angelica extract *BO*
Anise extract *BO*
Annatto extract *AD SS*
Apple extract *BO*
Apricot extract *BO*
Apricot kernel extract *BO*
Apricot kernel oil *CO EL*
Arachidyl alcohol *ES TK*
Arachidyl behenate *EL*
Argana oil *EL SS*
Arginine *CR*
Arnica extract (Arnica
  montana L.) *BO*
Artichoke extract *BO*
Asafoetida extract *BO*
Ascorbic acid *AO*
Ascorbyl oleate *AO*
Astragalus sinicus extract
  A
Atelocollagen *MO HU PT*
Avens extract *BO*
Avocado extract *BO*
Avocado oil *EL MO*
Avocado oil ethyl ester *EL*
Avocado oil
  unsaponifiables *EL*

Babassu oil *EL*
Babassuamidopropalk-
  onium chloride *FA*
Babassuamidopropyl
  betaine *FA*
Babassuamidopropyl-
  amine oxide *FA*
Balm mint extract *BO*
Balm mint oil *BO*
Banana extract *BO*
Barium sulfate *OP*

Barley extract *BO*
Basil extract *BO*
Batyl isostearate *EL*
Batyl stearate *EL*
Bay laurel extract *BO*
Bayberry wax *WX*
Bearberry extract *BO*
Bee pollen extract *BO*
Beeswax *ES*
Beet extract *BO*
Behenalkonium chloride
  CO
Behenamidopropyl
  dihydroxypropyl
  dimonium chloride
  CO EL ES
Behenamidopropyl PG
  dimonium chloride
  CO
Behenamidopropyldimeth-
  ylamine behenate *CO*
Behenamine oxide *CO FA*
Beheneth–5 *ES*
Beheneth–10 *ES*
Beheneth–20 *ES*
Beheneth–30 *ES*
Behenic acid *ES GE TK*
Behenoxy dimethicone *SI
  EL WX*
Behenoyl PG trimonium
  chloride *CO*
Behentrimonium chloride
  CO
Behenyl alcohol *EL TK*
Behenyl behenate *EL TK*
Behenyl betaine *CO ES*
Behenyl erucate *EL*
Behenyl isostearate *EL*
Behenylamidopropyl
  dimethylamine
  behenate *CO*
Behenylamidopropyl ethyl
  dimonium ethyl sulfate
  AS CO
Bentonite *SA TK TX*
Benzalkonium chloride
  AD AP
Benzoic acid *PR*
Benzophenone–1 *SS*
Benzophenone–2 *SS*
Benzophenone–3 *SS*
Benzophenone–4 *SS*
Benzophenone–6 *SS*

Benzophenone–8 *SS*
Benzophenone–9 *SS*
Benzophenone–11 *SS*
Benzophenone–12 *SS*
Benzyl laurate *EL*
Benzylparaben *PR*
Benzyltrimonium
  hydrolyzed collagen
  CO
BHA *AO*
BHT *AO*
Bilberry extract
  (Vaccinium mirtyllius
  L.) *BO*
Bioflavanoids *BO*
Birch leaf extract (Betula
  spp.) *BO*
Birchtree extract (Betula
  alba L.) *BO*
α-Bisabolol *AD*
bis-Diglyceryl-caprylate-
  caprate-isostearate-
  hydroxystearate-
  adipate *EL*
Bismuth oxychloride,
  coated mica *PE*
Bismuth oxychloride *PE*
Bitter orange extract *BO*
Bitter orange flowers
  extract *BO*
Bitter orange peel extract
  BO
Black cohosh extract *BO*
Blackcurrant extract *BO*
Black henna extract *BO*
Black walnut extract *BO*
Bladderwrack extract
  (Fucus vesiculosus L.)
  BO
Borage extract *BO*
Borage seed oil (Borago
  officinalis) *EL*
Boron nitride *LU*
Botanical extracts *BO*
Brain extract *EL*
Brazil nut oil *EL MO*
Bromochlorophene *AD*
Brucine sulfate *DN*
Buckthorn extract *BO*
Burdock extract (Arctium
  majus) *BO*
Burnet extract *BO*
Butane *PP*

Butcherbroom extract
(Ruscus aculeatus L.)
BO
Butyl acetate *SO*
Butyl methoxydibenzoyl-
methane *SS*
Butyl myristate *EL SO*
Butyl oleate *EL*
Butyl paraben sodium *PR*
Butyl stearate *EL SO*
Butylene glycol *SO*
Butyloctyl oleate *EL*
Butylparaben *PR*

C9–11 isoparaffin *SO*
C10–11 isoparaffin *SO*
C10–13 isoparaffin *SO*
C10–18 triglycerides *EL*
C10–30 cholestrol-
lanosterol esters *EL*
MO
C11–15 pareth–9 *SF*
C11–15 pareth–12 *SF*
C11–15 pareth–20 *SF*
C11–15 pareth–30 *SF*
C11–15 pareth–40 *SF*
C12 pareth carboxylic acid
SF
C12–13 alcohols *EL*
C12–13 pareth sulfate *SF*
C12–13 pareth–3 *ES*
C12–13 pareth–4 *ES*
C12–13 pareth–9 *ES*
C12–13 pareth–23 *ES*
C12–15 alcohols *TK*
C12–15 alcohols octanoate
EL
C12–15 alkyl benzoate *EL
SS*
C12–15 alkyl lactate *EL*
C12–15 linear alcohols 2-
ethyl-hexaonate *EL*
C12–15 pareth–12 *SF*
C12–16 alcohols *EL OP
TK*
C12–18 triglycerides *EL*
C12–C20 acid PEG–8 ester
ES
C14–15 alcohols *EL*
C14–15 pareth–8
carboxylic acid *SF*
C16–18 pareth–3 *ES*
C16–18 pareth–5.5 *ES*

C16–18 pareth–13 *ES*
C16–18 pareth–19 *ES*
C18–36 acid *TK*
C18–36 acid glycol ester
TK
C18–36 acidtriglyceride *TK*
C20–40 alcohol ethoclyate
SF
C20–40 alcohols *DS*
C30–50 alcohol ethoclyate
SF
C30–50 alcohols *DS*
C40–60 alcohol ethoclyate
SF
C40–60 alcohols *DS*
Cabbage rose extract *BO*
Calcium alginate *GE SA SB
TK*
Calcium carrageenan *TK*
Calcium disodium EDTA
CH
Calcium dodecylbenzene
sulfonate *ES SF*
Calcium laurate *SF*
Calcium protein complex
ES MO
Calcium stearate *LU*
Calcium stearoyl lactylate
ES HU
Calendula extract
(Calendula officinalis
L.) *BO*
Calendula oil *VA*
Camellia oil (Camellia
japonica) *EL GL*
Candelilla wax *WX*
Canola oil *EL*
Canolamidopropyl betaine
CO
Caper extract *BO*
Capramide DEA *CO DT ES*
Capryl caprylylglucoside
FA
Caprylic alcohol *SO TK*
Caprylic-capric acid *ES*
Caprylic-capric glycerides
ES
Caprylic-capric truglyceride
PEG–4 esters *EL*
Caprylic-capric-lauric
triglyceride *CO*
Caprylic-capric-linoleic
triglyceride *EL*

Caprylic-capric-oleis
triglycerides *CR*
Caprylic-capric-stearic
triglyceride *EL*
Caprylic-capric-succinic
triglyceride *EL*
Caprylic-capric-triglyceride
EL
Caprylic-capric-triglyceride
PEG–4 esters *EL*
Capryloamphogylcinate
AP FA
Capryloyl collagen amino
acids *AD*
Capryloyl glycine *AD*
Capryloyl keratin amino
acids *AD*
Caprylyl pyrrolidone *CO FA*
Capiscum extract *BO ST*
Capiscum oleoresin
(Capiscum frutescens
L.) *BO EL*
Captan *AD*
Carageenan extract *BO*
Caraway seed extract *BO*
Carbomer *TK*
Carboxymethyl
hydroxyethyl-cellulose
TK
Carnauba wax *WX*
Carrageenan *BO GE TK*
Carrageenan extract
(Chondrus crispus)
MO
Carrot extract (Daucus
carota L. var. Sativa)
BO
Carrot oil *BO*
Cashew oil *EL MO*
Castor oil, ethoxylated *ES*
Castor oil *DS EL SO*
Cebadilla extract *BO*
Celandine extract *BO*
Cellulose *TK*
Cellulose gum *SA TK*
Ceresin wax *GE WX*
Cetalkonium chloride *ES
WA*
Cetearalkonium chloride
CO
Cetaereth–2 *ES*
Cetaereth–2 phosphate *ES
SF*

Ceteareth–4 *ES*
Ceteareth–5 *ES*
Ceteareth–5 phosphate *ES
SF*
Ceteareth–6 *ES*
Ceteareth–8 *ES*
Ceteareth–10 *ES*
Ceteareth–10 phosphate
ES SF
Ceteareth–11 *ES*
Ceteareth–12 *ES*
Ceteareth–15 *ES*
Ceteareth–17 *ES*
Ceteareth–20 *ES*
Ceteareth–25 *ES*
Ceteareth–27 *ES*
Ceteareth–29 *ES*
Ceteareth–30 *ES*
Ceteareth–34 *ES*
Cetearyl alcohol *ES TK*
Cetearyl behenate *EL TK*
Cetearyl candelillate *EL GE*
Cetearyl glucoside *ES*
Cetearyl isononanoate *EL*
Cetearyl octanoate *EL OP
SO TK*
Cetearyl palmitate *EL*
Cetearyl stearate *EL TK*
Ceteth–2 *ES*
Ceteth–4 *ES*
Ceteth–6 *ES*
Ceteth–10 *EL ES*
Ceteth–12 *ES*
Ceteth–13 *ES*
Ceteth–16 *ES*
Ceteth–20 *ES*
Ceteth–25 *ES*
Ceteth–30 *ES*
Ceteth–33 *ES*
Cetethyldimonium
bromide *AD ES*
Cetethylmorphonlinium
ethosulfate *AS*
Cetoleth–25 *ES*
Cetostearyl stearate *EL TK*
Cetrimonium bromide *CO
PR*
Cetrimonium chloride *AS*
Cetyl acetate *EL*
Cetyl alcohol *EL TK*
Cetyl betaine *FA SF*
Cetyl C12–15 pareth–9
carboxylate *EL*

Cetyl caprylate *EL*
Cetyl dimethicone *WX*
Cetyl dimethicone
copolyol *ES*
Cetyl esters *EL*
Cetyl
hydroxyethylcellulose
SA TK
Cetyl isooctanoate *WX*
Cetyl lactate *EL*
Cetyl myristate *EL*
Cetyl octanoate *EL*
Cetyl oleate *EL*
Cetyl palmitate *EL TK*
Cetyl phosphate *ES SF*
Cetyl PPG–2 isodeceth–7
carboxylate *EL*
Cetyl pyridinium chloride
AD
Cetyl ricinoleate *EL*
Cetyl stearate *EL*
Cetyl stearyl octanoate *EL*
Chamomile extract,
English (Anthemis
nobilis) *BO*
Chamomile extract,
German (Matricaria
chamomila) *BO*
Chamomile oil, English
(Anthemis nobilis) *BO*
Chaulmoogra oil *VA*
Cherry pit oil *EL*
Chia oil (Salvia hispanica)
EL MO
Chitin, partially
deacetylated *FF HU*
Chitin *AS MO*
Chitosan *AS MO*
Chitosan lactate *FF*
Chitosan PCA *CO MO HU*
Chlorhexidine *AD*
Chlorhexidine diacetate
AD
Chlorhexidine
digluconate *AD*
Chlorhexidine
dihydrochloride *AD*
Chlorobutanol *SO*
Chlorophyllin copper
complex *DO*
Chlorothymol *AD*
Chloroxylenol *AD PR*
Chlorphenesin *AD PR*

Cholecalciferol *VT*
Cholestric esters *EL MO*
Cholesterol *EL ES MO*
Cholesteryl hydroxy
stearate *EL*
Cholesteryl stearate *EL*
Choleth–10 *ES*
Choleth–15 *ES*
Choleth–24 *EL ES*
Chondriotin sulfate *MO*
Cinchona extract
(Cinchona spp.) *BO*
Cinquefoil extract *BO*
Citric acid *CO*
Citroflavonoid, water
soluble *BO*
Citron oil *AD*
Citrus bioflavonoid
complex *BO*
Clove oil *AP*
Clover blossom extract *BO*
Cloves extract *BO*
Cocamide *FA TK*
Cocamide DEA *ES FA*
Cocamide MEA *FA TK*
Cocamide MIPA *FA RA TK*
Cocamidopropyl betaine,
potassium salt *SF*
Cocamidopropyl betaine
FA
Cocamidopropyl betaine
ammonium salt *SF*
Cocamidopropyl
dimethylamine
hydroxypropyl
hydrolyzed collagen *CO*
Cocamidopropyl
dimethylamine *CO ES
FA*
Cocamidopropyl
dimethylamine actate
DT
Cocamidopropyl
dimethylamine lactate
CO FA SB
Cocamidopropyl ethyl
dimonium ethosulfate
AS CO
Cocamidopropyl hydroxy
sultaine, ammonium
salt *SF*
Cocamidopropyl hydroxy
sultaine *FA*

Cocamidopropyl hydroxyl sultaine *FA*

Cocamidopropyl lauryl ether *FA OP*

Cocamidopropyl PG-dimonium chloride *CO EL*

Cocamidopropyl PG-dimonium chloride phosphate *CO ES*

Cocamidopropylamine oxide *FA SF TK*

Cocamidopropyldimonium hydroxypropylamino collagen *CO*

Cocamine *ES*

Cocamine oxide *FA SB*

Coceth–7 carboxylic acid *AD ES LU*

Cocomorpohline oxide *CO*

Coco rapeseedate *EL TK*

Coco-betaine *FA TK*

Coco-caprylate-caprate *EL*

Coco-hydrolyzed animal protein *PT*

Coco-hydrolyzed soy protein *EL SF*

Coco-oleamidopropyl betaine *CO FA TK*

Cocoa butter *EL*

Cocoamphodiacetate lauryl sulfate *SF*

Cocoamphodiacetate lauryl-laureth sulfate *SF*

Cocoamphodiacetate trideceth sulfate *SF*

Cocoamphodipropionate acid *WA*

Cocoamphoglycinate *DT FA*

Cocodimethyl betaine *DT FA*

Cocodimonium hydroxypropyl hydrolyzed collagen *CO PT*

Cocodimonium hydroxypropyl hydrolyzed hair keratin *CO*

Cocodimonium hydroxypropyl hydrolyzed soy protein *CO PT*

Coconut acid, potassium salt *FA*

Coconut acid *ES*

Coconut alcohol *CO*

Coconut oil *EL VA*

Cocoyl amido hydroxy sulfo betaine *FA TK*

Cocoyl midazoline *SF*

Cocoyl monoethanolamide ethoxylate *FA TK*

Cocoyl sarcosine *SF*

Coffee extract *SS*

Collagen *FF MO PT*

Collagen amino acids *CO MO*

Collagen amino-polysiloxane hydrolyzate *HU PT*

Collagen glycerides *CO*

Colloidal oatmeal *BO EL HU*

Colloidal silica sols *SB TK*

Coltsfoot extract (Tussilago farfara L.) *BO*

Comfrey extract *BO*

Coneflower extract (Echinacea spp) *AD BO*

Copper asparate *MO*

Copper disodium EDTA *CH*

Copper PCA *AD*

Copper PCA methylsilanol *HU*

Copper protein complex *ES MO*

Coriander extract *BO*

Corn Cob Powder *BO*

Corn oil *EL*

Corn poppy extract (Papaver rhoeas L.) *BO*

Corn soil extract *BO*

Cornflower extract (Centaurea cyranas L.) *BO*

Cornflower extract (Echinacea angustifolia Monch) *BO*

Cottonseed oil *EL*

Couch grass (Agropyron repens Beauv.) *BO*

Cranesbill extract *BO*

Crataegus extract (Crataegus oxyacantha Jacq.) *BO*

Crithumum maritimum *BO*

Cucumber extract (Cucumis sativus L.) *BO*

Cuttlefish extract *EL*

Cyclodextrins *CR ES SB*

Cyclohexane dimethanol dibezoate *PL*

Cyclomethicone *CO EL LU*

Cypress extract *BO*

d-Panthenyl triacetate *EL VT*

Dandelion extract (Taraxacum officinalis Weber) *BO*

Date extract *BO*

DEA lauryl sulfate *DT FA*

DEA-C21-dicarboxylate *ES*

DEA-ceteareth–2-phosphate *ES*

DEA-cetyl phosphate *ES*

DEA-hydrolyzed lecithin *FA TK*

DEA-laureth sulfate *FA*

DEA-linoleate *TK*

DEA-methoxycinnamate *SS*

DEA-oleth–3 phosphate *ES TK*

DEA-oleth–5 phosphate *ES SF*

DEA-oleth–10 phosphate *ES*

DEA-oleth–20 phosphate *ES SF*

Dead Sea mud *BO*

Dead Sea Salts *BO*

Decaglyceryl pentastearate *ES*

Decamethyl cyclopentasiloxane *CR EL*
Deceth–3 *SF*
Deceth–4 phosphate *EL*
Deceth–6 *SF*
Deceth–8 *SF*
Deceth–9 *WA*
Declytetraddeceth–25 *DT*
Decyl alcohol *SO TK*
Decyl oleate *EL*
Decyl polyglucose *FA*
Decyl tetradecanol *EL*
Decylglucoside *FA*
Decyltetradeceth–25 *SF*
Denatonium benzoate *DN*
Denatonium saccharide *DN*
Deoxy ribonucleic acid *PT*
Desamido collagen *FF MO*
Dextran *TK*
Dextrin *TK*
Di-lauryl acetyl dinonium chloride *CO ES*
Di-octyldodeceth–2 lauroyl glutamate *SF*
Di-octyldodecyl lauroyl glutamate *SF*
Di-steareth–2 lauroyl glutamate *SF*
Di-steareth–5 lauroyl glutamate *SF*
Dialkyldimethypolysil-oxane *EL WX*
Diamyl sodium sulfosuccinate *DT*
Diazolidinyl urea *PR*
Dibehenyl-diarachidyl dimonium chloride *CO*
Dibehenyldimonium chloride *CO*
Dibenzylidene sorbitol *GE MO*
Dibutyl phthalate *PL*
Dibutyl sebacate *EL*
Dicapryl adipate *EL*
Diceteareth–10 phosphoric acid *ES SF*
Dichlorobenzyl alcohol *AD AP PR*
Dichlorophene *PR*

Dicoco distearyl pentaerythrityl citrate *ES*
Dicyclohexyl sodium sulfosuccinate *DT*
Didecyldimonium chloride *AP CO*
Diethyl phthalate *PL*
Diethyl sebacate *SO*
Diethylaminoethyl stearate *ES*
Diethylene glycol *SO*
Diethylene glycol dibenzoate *SO PL*
Diethylene glycol diisononanoate *EL*
Diethylene glycol diotanoate *EL*
Diethylene glycol stearyl oxide *ES*
Difluoroethane *PP*
Diglyceryl dioleate *GL SF SO*
Diglyceryl monoisostearate *GL SF SO*
Diglyceryl stearate malate *ES*
Diglyceryl triisostearate *OP SF SO*
Dihydroabietyl behenate *EL*
Dihydrocholeth–15 *ES*
Dihydrocholeth–20 *ES*
Dihydrocholeth–30 *ES*
Dihydrogenated tallow phthalic acid amide *SA*
Dihydroxyethyl C12–15 alkoxypropylamine oxide *FA*
Dihydroxyethyl cocamine oxide *CO FA*
Dihydroxyethyl dihydroxy-propyl stearmonium chloride *CO*
Dihydroxyethyl tallowamine oleate *EL*
Dihydroxyethyl tallow glycinate *CO*
Dihydroxyethyl tallowamine oxide *FA CO*
Diisobutyl adipate *EL*

Diisobutyl sodium sulfosuccinate *DT*
Diisocetyl adipate *EL SO*
Diisopropyl adipate *EL SO*
Diisopropyl dilinoleate *EL*
Diisopopryl dimer dilinoleate *EL*
Diisopropyl sebacate *EL SO*
Diisostearyl adipate *EL*
Diisostearyl dimer dilinoleate *AD EL*
Diisostearyl fumarate *EL*
Diisostearyl malate *EL*
Diistearyl fumarate *LU*
Dilaureth–10 phosphate *TK*
Dilauryldimonium chloride *AD*
Dilinoleamidopropyl dimethylamine *CO*
Dilinoleamidopropyl dimethylamine dimethicone copolyol phosphate *ES*
Dilinoleic acid *EL ES*
Dimethicone *EL LU SI*
Dimethicone copolyol *LU SF SI*
Dimethicone copolyol phosphate *ES*
Dimethicone propyl PG-betaine *SF*
Dimethicone propylethylenediamine behenate *EL*
Dimethyl behenamine *AS*
Dimethyl cocamine *AS*
Dimethyl ether *PP*
Dimethyl hyalauronate *MO*
Dimethyl hydrogenated tallowamine *CO*
Dimethyl hydroxy methyl pyrazole *PR*
Dimethyl lauramine *CO FA*
Dimethyl lauramine isostearate *CO*
Dimethyl myristamine *CO*
Dimethyl oxazolidine *PR*
Dimethyl palmitamine *AS*
Dimethyl phthalate *PL SO*
Dimethyl soyamine *AS CO*

Dimethyl stearamine *CO*
Dimethyl tallowamine *AS*
Dimethylamidopropyl-
amine dimearate *CO*
Dimethylsilanol
hyaluronate *MO*
Dioctyl adipate *EL*
Dioctyl dimer dilinoleate
EL
Dioctyl malate *EL*
Dioctyl maleate *MO*
Dioctyl sebacate *EL*
Dioctyl sodium
sulfosuccinate *WA*
Dioctyl succinate *EL*
Dioctylcyclohexane *EL*
Dioctyldodeceth–5 lauroyl
glutamate *SF*
Dioleth–8 phosphate *TK*
Dipalmitoyl cystine *AD*
Dipalmitoylethyl
hydroxyethylmonium
methosulfate *CO*
Dipentaerythritol fatty
acid ester *EL MO*
Dipentaerythrityl
hexacapratehexacapry-
late *EL*
Dipentaethylthrite
hexahydroxy-stearate-
isostearate *EL*
Diphenyl dimethicone
GL
Dipotassium
glycyrrhizinate *AD HU*
Dipropylene glycol *ES SO*
Dipropylene glycol
dibenzoate *SO PL*
Disodium
caproamphodiacetate
DT FA
Disodium
caproamphodipropion-
ate *DT FA*
Disodium
caprylamphodiacetate
DT
Disodium
caprylamphodipropion-
ate *DT*
Disodium
capryloamphodiace-
tate *FA SF*

Disodium cetearyl
sulfosuccinate *DT*
Disodium cocamido MEA-
sulfosuccinate *DT FA*
Disodium cocamido MIPA-
sulfosuccinate *DT*
Disodium
cocoamphodiacetate
FA SF
Disodium
cocoamphodiprop-
ionate *DT FA*
Disodium deceth–6
sulfosuccinate *DT*
Disodium EDTA *AO CH
PR*
Disodium hydrogenated
cottonseed glyceride
sulfosuccinate *CO ES*
Disodium hydrogenated
tallow glutamate *SF*
Disodium isodecyl
sulfosuccinate *DT*
Disodium laneth–5
sulfosuccinate *SF*
Disodium lauramido MEA
sulfosuccinate *DT FA SF*
Disodium lauramido
PEG–2 sulfosuccinate
DT
Disodium laureth
sulfosuccinate *CO DT
FA SF*
Disodium
lauroamphodiacetate
CO FA
Disodium
lauroamphodiprop-
ionate *DT FA*
Disodium lauryl
sulfosuccinate *DT*
Disodium myristamido
MEA-sulfosuccinate
DT
Disodium nonoxynol–10
sulfosuccinate *FA*
Disodium oleamido MEA
sulfosuccinate *FA*
Disodium oleamido MIPA
sulfosuccinate *FA SF*
Disodium oleamido
PEG–2 sulfosuccinate
DT

Disodium PEG–4
cocoamido MIPA
sulfosuccinate *DT FA*
Disodium ricinoleamido
MEA sulfosuccinate
DT ES SF
Disodium stearyl
sulfosuccinate *ES*
Disodium tallamido MEA
sulfosuccinate *SF*
Disodium
tallowiminodiprop-
ionate *DT*
Disodium
undecylenamido MEA
sulfosuccinate *AD*
Disodium-PG-
propyldimethicone
thiosulfate *SI*
Distearyldimethylamine
dilinoleate *EL*
Distearyldimonium
chloride *CO*
Ditridecyl adipate *EL*
dl–C12–15 Alkyl fumarate
EL
DMDM hydantoin *PR*
DMHF *FF TK*
Dodecylphenol-ethylene
oxide condensate *ES*
Dodoxynol–6 *DT*
Dodoxynol–9 *DT*
Domiphen bromide *AD*
Drometrizole *SS*
Dyper's broom extract *BO*

EDTA *AO CH PR*
Egg Yolk extract *EL ES*
Elastin amino acids *MO
PT*
Elder extract (Sambucus
nigra L.) *BO*
Elderflower extract *BO*
Elderflower oil *A*
Elderberry extract *BO*
Eleuthero ginseng extract
BO ST
Elm bark extract *BO*
Embryo extract *PT*
Emulsifying wax *ES WX*
Ergocalciferol *VT*
Erucyl erucate *EL*
Esculin *VT*

Ethanolamine HCI *BF*
Ethyl acetate *SO*
Ethyl avocadate *EL*
Ethyl dihydroxypropyl
  PABA *SS*
Ethyl ester of hydrolyzed
  collagen *CO PT*
Ethyl ester of hydrolyzed
  silk *FF HU*
Ethyl hexanediol *ES*
Ethyl hydrolyzed keratin
  protein *PT*
Ethyl hydroxymethyl oleyl
  oxazoline *DS WA*
Ethyl lactate *SO*
Ethyl linoleate *VT*
Ethyl linolenate *EL*
Ethyl minkate *EL MO*
Ethyl morrhuate *EL*
Ethyl myristate *EL SO*
Ethyl oleate *EL SO*
Ethyl olivate *EL*
Ethyl panthenol *MO*
Ethyl paraben sodium *PR*
Ethyl salicylate *SS*
Ethylcellulose *FF*
Ethylene glycol phenyl
  ether *PR*
Ethylene glycol stearate *ES*
  OP PE
Ethylene vinyl acetate *RS*
Ethylene vinyl alcohol *RS*
Ethylene-acrylic acid
  copolymer *GE*
Ethylene-vinyl acetate
  copolymer *GE*
Ethylhexyl isopalmitate *EL*
Ethylparaben *PR*
Etocrylene *SS*
Eucalyptus extract
  (Eucalyptus globulus
  Labill.) *BO*
Eucalyptus oil *BO*
Euglena gracillis
  polysaccharide *ES*
Euphrasia extract *BO*
Evening primrose oil
  (Oenothera spp) *EL*
  MO
Everlasting extract *BO*

Fatty alcohol, C12–15
  sulfate, sodium salt *FA*

Fatty quarternary amine
  chloride complex *HU*
Fennel extract *BO*
Fenugreek extract
  (Trigonella foenum-
  graecum L.) *BO*
Fern extract *BO*
Ferulic acid *AO*
Fibronectin *PT*
Fig extract *BO*
Fir needle extract *BO*
Formaldehyde *PR*
Fucales *BO*
Fumitory extract (Fumaria
  officinalis L.) *BO*

Gardenia extract *BO*
Garlic extract *BO*
Gelatin *FF PT*
Gellan gum *FF GE SB TK*
Gentian extract
  (Gentriana lutea L.)
  BO
Geranium extract *BO*
Ginkgo biloba extract
  (Gingko biloba L.)
Ginseng extract (Panax
  ginseng C.A. Meyer)
  BO
Glechoma hederacea
  extract *BO*
Glucose glutamate *HU*
Glutaral *PR*
Glycereth–4,5-lactate *HU*
Glycereth–5 lactate *HU*
Glycereth–7 *HU*
Glycereth–7 benzoate *EL*
Glycereth–7
  diisononanoate *EL*
Glycereth–7 triacetate *EL*
Glycereth–7 trioctanate *EL*
Glycereth–12 *EL MO HU*
Glycereth–25 PCA
  isostearate *SF*
Glycereth–26 *EL HU*
Glycereth–26 phosphate
  ES SF
Glycerin *HU*
Glycerol tribenzoate *PL*
Glycerol tricaprylate-
  caprate *EL*
Glyceryl abietate *RS*
Glyceryl adipate *EL*

Glyceryl behenate *TK*
Glyceryl caprylate *AD ES*
Glyceryl caprylate-caprate
  ES
Glyceryl citrate / lactate /
  lioleate / oleate *ES*
Glyceryl cocoate *ES*
Glyceryl diisostearate *DS SB*
Glyceryl dilaurate *ES*
Glyceryl dioleate *EL ES*
Glyceryl distearate *ES OP*
Glyceryl hydroxystearate
  ES OP SF
Glyceryl isostearate *EL ES*
  LU
Glyceryl lanolate *EL ES*
Glyceryl laurate *AD PR*
Glyceryl linoleate *EL ES*
Glyceryl mono
  undecylenate *ES*
Glyceryl mono-di-tri-
  caprylate *ES SB*
Glyceryl
  monopyroglutamate
  AS EL
Glyceryl myristate *EL ES*
  OP
Glyceryl oleate *EL ES LU*
Glyceryl PABA *SS*
Glyceryl palmitate *ES*
Glyceryl ricinoleate *EL ES*
Glyceryl stearate *ES OP TK*
Glyceryl stearate citrate *ES*
Glyceryl stearate lactate *ES*
Glyceryl stearate SE *ES SB*
Glyceryl triacetyl
  hydroxystearate *EL*
Glyceryl triacetyl
  ricinoleate *EL*
Glycine *BF CO*
Glycofurol *SO*
Glycol *PL*
Glycol distearate *OP PE*
Glycol oleate *ES*
Glycol palmitate *ES*
Glycol stearate SE *ES PE*
Glycolamide stearate *ES*
  PE
Glycoproteins *CO*
Glycosaminoglycans *EL*
  MO
Glycosphingolipids *EL ES*
  MO

Glycyrrhetinic acid BO
Glycyrrhizic acid BO
Glycyrrhizin, ammoniated BO
Grape extract BO
Grape leaf extract (Vitis palmata) BO
Grape seed extract BO
Grape seed oil EL
Grape skin extract BO
Grapefruit extract (Citrus paradisi) BO
Green bean extract BO
Guaiazulene AD
Guanine PE
Guar gum SA TK
Guar hydroxypropyltrimonium chloride BO ST
Guarana extract BO ST
Gum karaya CO FF

Harpagophytum extract (Harpagophytum procumbens D.C.) BO
Hawaiian ginger extract BO
Hayflower extract BO
Hazlenut extract BO
Hazlenut oil EL
Hectorite SA TK TX
HEDTA AO CH PR
Henna extract (Lawsonia inermis) BO CO
Hesperidin complexes BO
Hesperidin methyl chalcone BO
Hexachlorophene AP
Hexadecyl isopalmitate EL
Hexahydro 1,3,5 tris (2-hydroxyet)-5-triazine PR
Hexamethyldisiloxane EL
Hexamidine diisethionate AD PR
Hexanediol behenyl beeswax GE
Hexetidine AD
Hexyl alcohol SO TK
Hexyl laurate EL
Hexyldecanol EL
Hibiscus extract (Hisbiscus sabdariffa) BO
Hinokitiol AD

Homosalate SS
Honey extract EL MO HU
Honey melon extract BO
Honeysuckle extract (Lonicera caprifolium) BO A AD
Hops extract (Humulus lupulus L.) A BO
Horse chestnut extract (Aesculus hippocstanum L.) BO
Horseradish extract (Cochlearia armoracia) BO
Horsetail extract (Equisetum arvense L.) BO
Human placental protein PT
Hyaluronic acid MO LU
Hyacinth extract BO
Hybrid safflower oil EL MO
Hydrated silica TK
Hydrocotyl extract BO
Hydrocotyl extract (Centella asiatica L.) BO
Hydrogenated C6-C14 olefin polymers EL
Hydrogenated castor oil DS EL WX
Hydrogenated castor oil laurate EL
Hydrogenated coco-glycerides ES SB
Hydrogenated coconut oil EL
Hydrogenated cottonseed oil EL
Hydrogenated jojoba wax GE
Hydrogenated lanolin, distilled EL
Hydrogenated lanolin EL ES
Hydrogenated lecithin DS ES MO
Hydrogenated milk fat EL
Hydrogenated mink oil EL
Hydrogenated palm kernel glycerides EL RA

Hydrogenated palm oil EL
Hydrogenated passion fruit oil HU
Hydrogenated polyisobutene EL MO
Hydrogenated rapeseed oil TK WX
Hydrogenated rice bran wax WX
Hydrogenated soybean oil EL
Hydrogenated starch hydrolysate EL TK
Hydrogenated tallow amine oxide AS CO
Hydrogenated tallow glyceride DS EL ES SB
Hydrogenated tallow glyceride lactate EL
Hydrogenated tallow glycerides citrate ES
Hydrogenated tallowtrimonium chloride CO
Hydrogenated turtle oil EL
Hydrogenated vegetable glycerides EL
Hydrogenated vegetable oil EL VA WX
Hydrolyzed conchiolin protein CO EL
Hydrolyzed elastin MO
Hydrolyzed extensin CO PT
Hydrolyzed fibronectin CO MO HU
Hydrolyzed fish protein CO PT
Hydrolyzed glycosaminoglycans MO
Hydrolyzed hemoglobin PT
Hydrolyzed keratin CO EL FF MO PT
Hydrolyzed mild protein CO PT
Hydrolyzed oat protein BO EL HU
Hydrolyzed placental protein MO
Hydrolyzed reticulin CO

Hydrolyzed RNA *FF*
Hydrolyzed serum protein *MO*
Hydrolyzed silk *CO FF MO*
Hydrolyzed soy protein *CO FF PT*
Hydrolyzed vegetable protein *PT*
Hydrolyzed wheat protein *FA MO PT*
Hydrolyzed wheat protein polysiloxane polymer *CO*
Hydrolyzed wheat protein-dimethicone copolyol phosphate copolymer *FF*
Hydrolyzed zein *FX*
Hydroquinone *AO*
Hydroxycetyl hydroxyethyl dimonium chloride *CO*
Hydroxycetyl phosphate *ES*
Hydroxyethycellulose *TK*
Hyddroxyethyl stearamide-MIPA *PE*
Hydroxylated lanolin *EL ES*
Hydroxylated lecithin *ES*
Hydroxylated milk glyceride *EL*
Hydroxyoctacosanyl hydroxystearate *ES SB*
Hydroxyproline *CO*
Hydroxypropyl bisstearyldimonium chloride *CO*
Hydroxypropyl chitosan *CO TK*
Hydroxypropyl guar *LU TK*
Hydroxypropyl guar hydroxypropyl trimonium chloride *CO*
Hydroxypropyl methylcellulose *FA TK*
Hydroxypropyl-bisisostearyamidopropyldimonium chloride *CO ES*
Hydroxypropylcellulose *FF TK*

Hydroxypropyltrimonium hydrolyzed keratin *CO*
Hydroxypropyltrimonium hydrolyzed silk *CO*
Hydroxypropyltrimonium wheat protein *CO*
Hydroxystearic acid *EL GE*
Hypericum extract *BO*

I-Gluatmic acid *CO*
Iceland moss extract *AD*
Illipe butter *EL*
Imidazolidinyl urea *PR*
Indian cress extract (Tropaeolum majus L.) *BO*
Inositol *MO*
Isoamyl p-methoxycinnamate *SS*
Isobutane *PP*
Isobutyl palmitate *EL*
Isobutyl stearate *EL SO*
Isobutylene-maleic anhydride copolymer *DS SA*
Isobutylparaben *PR*
Isoceteareath–8 stearate *ES*
Isoceteth–10 *TK*
Isoceteth–10 stearate *ES*
Isoceteth–20 *ES*
Isocetyl alcohol *DS ES*
Isocetyl behenate *EL*
Isocetyl octanoate *EL*
Isocetyl palmitate *EL*
Isocetyl salicylate *EL SO*
Isocetyl stearate *EL*
Isodecyl benzoate *PL SO*
Isodecyl citrate *EL*
Isodecyl cocoate *EL*
Isodecyl hydroxypropanetricar-boxylic acid *EL*
Isodecyl isononanoate *EL*
Isodecyl laurate *EL*
Isodecyl neopentanoate *EL*
Isodecyl octanoate *EL*
Isodecyl oleate *EL SO*
Isodecyl salicylate *EL ST*
Isodecyl stearate *EL LU*
Isododecane *SO*
Isoeicosane *EL GL*
Isohexadecane *EL SO*

Isolaureth–6 *ES WA*
Isononyl isononanoate *EL*
Isooctadecyl hexadecanoate *EL*
Isooctadecyl isononanoate *WX*
Isopentacontaoctacane *EL GL*
Isopentyldiol *EL*
Isopropanolamine lauryl sulfate *FA DT*
Isopropyl alcohol *SO*
Isopropyl avocadate *EL*
Isopropyl C12–15 pareth–9-carboxylate *EL*
Isopropyl isostearate *EL*
Isopropyl lanolate *EL LU PL*
Isopropyl linoleate *EL*
Isopropyl methoxycinnamate *SS*
Isopropyl myristate *EL SO*
Isopropyl palmitate *EL SO*
Isopropyl paraben *PR*
Isopropyl PPG–2-isodeceth–7 carboxylate *EL*
Isopropyl sorbate *PR*
Isopropyl stearate *EL*
Isopropylamine dodecyl benzenesulfonate *DT*
Isopropylbenzylsalicylate *SS*
Isosorbide laurate *EL*
Isostearamide DEA *FA TK*
Isostearamido propyl dimethylamine *AS CO*
Isostearamidopropyl betaine *CO DT*
Isostearamidopropyl dimethylamine gluconate *CO ES*
Isostearamidopropyl dimethylamine glycolate *CO ES*
Isostearamidopropyl dimethylamine lactate *CO*
Isostearamidopropyl ethyldimonium ethosulfate *CO*

Isostearamidopropyl lanurylacetodimonium chloride *CO ES*
Isostearamidopropyl morpholine *CO*
Isostearamidopropyl morpholine lactate *CO*
Isostearamidopropyl morpholine oxide *CO*
Isostearamidopropyl dimonium chloride *CO*
Isostearamidopropylamide oxide *FA TK*
Isostearamidopropylkonium chloride *CO*
Isosteareth–2 *ES*
Isosteareth–2-octanoate *ES*
Isosteareth–3 *ES*
Isosteareth–6 carboxylic acid *DT*
Isosteareth–10 *ES*
Isosteareth–10 stearate *ES*
Isosteareth–12 *ES*
Isosteareth–20 *ES*
Isosteareth–22 *ES*
Isosteareth–50 *ES*
Isostearic acid *EL ES*
Isostearoamphopropionate *DT TK*
Isostearoyl hydrolyzed collagen *CO PL PT*
Isostearyl alcohol *EL*
Isostearyl behenate *EL*
Isostearyl benzoate *EL*
Isostearyl diglyceryl succinate *EL ES LU*
Isostearyl erucate *EL*
Isostearyl erucyl erucate *EL*
Isostearyl hydrolyzed animal protein *CO MO*
Isostearyl imidazoline *DT*
Isostearyl isostearate *EL RA*
Isostearyl lactate *EL*
Isostearyl malate *EL*
Isostearyl myristate *EL*
Isostearyl neopentanoate *EL*
Isostearyl palmitate *EL*
Isostearyl stearoyl stearate *SO EL*

Isostearylamidopropyl dihydroxypropyl dimonium chloride *CO EL ES*
Isotridecyl cocoate *EL*
Isotridecyl isononanoate *EL*
Isotridecyl myristate *EL*
Ivy extract (Hedera helix L.) *BO*

Japan wax *WX*
Jasmine extract (Jasminum officinale) *BO*
Job's tears extract *SS*
Jojoba butter *EL*
Jojoba esters *EL MO WX*
Jojoba oil, synthetic *EL*
Jojoba oil *BO MO*
Jojoba wax *GE TK*
Jujube extract *AD*
Juniper extract (Jupierus communis L.) *BO*

Kalaya oil *EL*
Karaya gum *TK*
Kelp extract *BO*
Keratin *PT*
Keratin amino acids *MO*
Kiwi extract *MO*
Kiwi oil *BO*
Kola nut extract *BO*
Konjac mannan *BO MO*
Krameria extract (Krameria tiandra Ruiz et Pav.) *BO*
Kukui nut oil *EL*

Lactalbumin hydrolysate *CO PT*
Lactamide DGA *EL*
Lactamide MEA *MO HU*
Lactamidopropyl trimonium chloride *HU*
Lactic acid *HU*
Lactic acid monoethanolamide *EL LU*
Lactococcus hydrolysate *MO ST*

β–Lactoglobolin *CO FF PT*
Lactoyl methylsilnol elastinate *MO*
Lady's mantle extract (Silybum marignum) *BO*
Laneth–5 *ES GE*
Laneth–10 *ES*
Laneth–15 *ES GE*
Laneth–16 *ES*
Laneth–20 *ES*
Laneth–40 *ES*
Lanolin *EL ES*
Lanolin acid *DS EL WA*
Lanolin alcohol *EL ES MO*
Lanolin fatty acids *ES*
Lanolin oil *EL LU*
Lanolin wax *ES*
Lanosterol *EL*
Laramide DEA *FA*
Laramide MEA *FA*
Lard glyceride *EL*
Lauralkonium bromide *AD*
Lauralkonium chloride *AD*
Lauramide DEA *ES TK*
Lauramide MEA *TK*
Lauramide MIPA *FA TK*
Lauramidopropyl betaine *FA SF TK*
Lauramidopropyl dimethylamine *CO ES*
Lauramidopropyl PG-dimonium chloride *CO ES*
Lauramidopropyl PG-dimonium chloride phosphate *CO*
Lauromidopropylamine oxide *DT FA*
Lauramine oxide *CO FA*
Lauramine PG-glycinate phosphate *CO*
Laurel extract *BO*
Laureth carboxylic acid *SF*
Laureth–1 *ES SF*
Laureth–2 *EL ES SF*
Laureth–2 acetate *EL*
Laureth–2 benzoate *EL*
Laureth–2 octanoate *EL ES*

Laureth–3 *EL ES SB SF*

Laureth–3 carboxylic acid *SF*

Laureth–3 phosphate *ES LU SF*

Laureth–4 *DS ES SF*

Laureth–4 carboxylic acid *ES*

Laureth–5 *ES*

Laureth–5 carboxylic acid *ES SF*

Laureth–6 *DS ES*

Laureth–7 *ES SF*

Laureth–9 *ES*

Laureth–10 *FA TK*

Laureth–11 *DT ES SF*

Laureth–11 carboxylic acid *ES*

Laureth–12 *ES SF*

Laureth–16 *DS ES SF*

Laureth–20 *ES*

Laureth–23 *ES*

Laureth–25 *ES*

Laureth–30 *ES*

Lauric-linoleic DEA *FA TK*

Lauroampho PG-glycinate phosphate *DT*

Lauroyl collagen amino acids *AD*

Lauroyl hydrolyzed collagen *CO PL*

Lauroyl lysine *HU*

Lauroyl sarcosine *SF*

Lauroyl-linoleoyl diethanolamide *FA TK*

Lauroyl-myristoyl diethanolamide *FA TK*

Laurtrimonium chloride *AD CO*

Lauryl alcohol *TK*

Lauryl betaine *FA TK*

Lauryl dimethylamine C21-dicarboxylate *SF*

Lauryl hydroxyethyl imidazoline *SF*

Lauryl lactate *EL*

Lauryl methyl gluceth–10 hydroxypropyldimonium chloride *CO*

Lauryl PCA *ES MO*

Lauryl phosphate *CO DT EL*

Lauryl polyglucose *FA*

Lauryl pyrrolidone *CO FA WA*

Lauryldimethylamine isostearate *EL*

Lauryldimethylamine oleate *EL*

Lauryldimonium hydrolyzed animal protein *CO*

Lauryldimonium hydroxypropyl hydrolyzed collagen *AS CO PT*

Lauryldimonium hydroxypropyl hydrolyzed keratin *CO*

Lauryldimonium hydroxypropyl hydrolyzed soy protein *CO*

Laurylmethicone copolyol *ES*

Laurylpyridinium chloride *AD*

Lavender extract (Lavandula officinalis) *BO*

LEA iodine *BO*

Lecithin *CO ES MO RA WA*

Lecithin modified kaolin *OP*

Lecithin modified mica *PE*

Lemon balm (Melissa officinalis L.) *BO*

Lemon extract (Citrus limonum R.) *A BO*

Lemongrass extract *BO*

Lesquerella oil *EL MO*

Lettuce extract *BO*

Lichen extract *AD*

Licorice extract *AD BO*

Lilac extract *BO*

Lily extract (Lilium candidum L.) *BO*

Linden extract (Tilia spp.) *BO*

Linol linolenic acid *CO*

Linoleamide DEA *RA SF TK FA*

Linoleamidepropyl PG-dimonium chloride phosphate *ES*

Linoleamidepropyldim-ethylamine *CO*

Linoleamidepropyldim-ethylamine dimer dilinoleate *AS*

Linoleic acid *EL TK*

Liposomes *CR MO RA*

Lithium stearates *ES*

Lithothamnum calcareum *BO*

Live yeast cell derivative *MO*

Live yeast cell derivative liposome *CR*

Locust bean gum *TK*

Lysine PCA *AO MO*

Macadamia nut oil *EL*

Madder (Rubia tinctorum L.) *BO*

Magnesium aluminium silicate *SA TK*

Magnesium aspartate *MO*

Magnesium laureth sulfate *DT*

Magnesium laureth–8 sulfate *SF*

Magnesium lauryl sulfate *DT*

Magnesium myristate *LU*

Magnesium PEG–3 cocamide sulfate *DT*

Magnesium stearate *LU*

Magnesium sulfate heptahydrate (epsom salt) *ES RA*

Maleated soybean oil *EL ES*

Malic acid *CH*

Mallow extract (Malva sylvestris L.) *BO*

Maltitol *MO SB*

Mandragora extract *BO*

Manganese asparate *MO*

Mango extract *EL*

Mannitol *HU*

Marine polyamino-accharide *MO*

MDM hydantoin *PR TK*

MEA-dodecylbenzene-sulfonate *DT*

MEA-laureth sulfate *DT ES FA*

MEA-lauryl sulfate *DT SF*
Meadowsweet extract *BO*
Melaleuca oil *VA*
Melanin *AO DS*
Menthyl anthranilate *SS*
Meroxapol 105 *SF*
Meroxapol 171 *SF*
Meroxapol 172 *SF*
Methcrylol ethyl bethainemethacrylates copolymer *RS*
Methene ammonium chloride *PR*
Methicone *SI*
Methoxy PEG–17 dedecyl glycol copolymer *ES*
Methoxydiglycol *SO*
Methoxyisopropanol *SO*
Methyl acetyl ricinoleate *EL*
Methyl gallate *AO*
Methyl gluceth–10 *GL HU*
Methyl gluceth–20 *FA HU*
Methyl gluceth–20 benzoate *EL*
Methyl gluceth–20 distearate *EL ES*
Methyl glucose dioleate *ES*
Methyl glucose sesquiisostearate *ES*
Methyl glucose sesquisteate *EL*
Methyl hydroxystearate *EL*
Methyl paraben sodium *PR*
Methyl ricinoleate *EL*
Methyl rosinate *FX*
Methyl salicylate *AP*
Methylated cyclodextrin *SB*
Methylcellulose *TK*
Methyldibromo glutaronitrile *PR*
Methylene chloride *SO*
Methylparaben *PR*
Methylsilanol elastinate *MO PT ST*
Methylsilanol hydroxyproline aspartate *ST*
Methylsilanol mannuronate *MO*
Mexican poppy oil *VA*

Mica *PE*
Microcrystalline wax *EL*
Milk protein *CO*
Mineral oil *EL MO LU*
Mink oil *EL LU*
Mink wax *ES*
Mistletoe extract *BO*
Mixed isopropanolamines myristate *FA SF*
Mixed mucopolysaccharides *EL*
Molybdenum aspartate *MO*
Monostearyl citrate *CH PL*
Montan wax *WX*
Montmorillonite *TK*
Morpholine *SO*
Mulberry extract *AD*
Mushroom extract *BO*
Musk rose oil *EL*
Myreth–3 *CA EL ES*
Myreth–3 caprate *EL*
Myreth–3 myristate *EL ES*
Myreth–3 octanoate *EL GE*
Myreth–4 *ES*
Myreth–7 *ES SF*
Myrrh extract (Commiphora myrra Nees) *BO*
Myristalkonium chloride *AD CO*
Myristalkonium saccharinate *AD AP*
Myristamide DEA *FA TK*
Myristamide MEA *FA TK*
Myristamide oxide *TK*
Myristamidopropyl betaine *CO*
Myristamidopropyl dimethylamine *CO ES*
Myristamidopropyl dimethylamine dimethicone copolyol phosphate *FA*
Myristamine oxide *DT FA*
Myristic acid *DT*
Myristoyl hydrolyzed collagen *FF*
Myristoyl sarcosine *SF*
Myristyl alcohol *EL SF TK*
Myristyl myristate *EL*

Myristyl octanoate *EL*
Myristyl propionate *EL*
Myristyl stearate *EL*
Myrtrimonium bromide *CO PR*

N,N,N',N'-Tetrakis(2-hydroxypropyl)ethyl-enediamine *CH*
/N,O/-Carboxymethyl chitin *AS*
N,O-Carboxymethyl-chitosan *FF GE*
N,O-Carboxymethyl-chitosoniumn *FF GE*
n-Butyl alcohol *SO*
N-Cocoyl-(3-amidopropyl)-N,N-dimethyl-N-ethyl ammonium ethyl sulfate *SF*
N-Ethylether-bis–1,4-(N-isostearylamidopropyl-N,N-dimethyl ammonium *CO ES*
Nasturtium extract *BO*
Natto gum *HU*
Neatsfoot oil *EL LU*
Neem oil *EL*
Neopentyl glucol dibenzoate *PL*
Neopentyl glycol dicaprate *EL MO*
Neopentyl glycol dioctanoate *EL*
Neopentylglycol dicapratedicaprylate *EL*
Neopentylglycol diisooctanoate *EL*
Neroli extract *BO*
Nettle extract *BO*
Niacinamide *VT*
Nicotine sulfate *DN*
Nitrocellulose *FF*
Nonoxynol–1 *ES*
Nonoxynol–2 *DS ES*
Nonoxynol–4 *ES*
Nonoxynol–5 *ES*
Nonoxynol–6 *ES*
Nonoxynol–7 *ES SF*
Nonoxynol–8 *ES*
Nonoxynol–9 *ES SF*
Nonoxynol–10 *DT ES*

Nonoxynol–10 carboxylic acid *SF*
Nonoxynol–11 *ES*
Nonoxynol–12 *ES*
Nonoxynol–13 *ES SF*
Nonoxynol–14 *ES*
Nonoxynol–15 *ES SF*
Nonoxynol–18 *DS ES*
Nonoxynol–20 *DS ES*
Nonoxynol–30 *DS ES*
Nonoxynol–40 *DS ES*
Nonoxynol–50 *DS ES*
Nonoxynol–50 *ES*
Nonyl nonoxynol–5 *ES WA*
Nonyl nonoxynol–10 *ES*
Nordihydroguaiaretic acid *AO*
Nymphaeae alba root extract *BO*

o-Benzyl-p-chlorophenol *AP*
o-Cymen–5-ol *PR*
o-Phenylphenol *AD PR*
Oak bark extract *BO*
Oak root extract (Quercus) *BO*
Oak β–glucan *FF MO*
Oat extract (Avena sativa) *BO*
Oat flour *BO EL*
Oat protein *BO EL HU*
Octacosanyl stearate *EL GE TK*
Octamethyl cyclotetrasiloxane *SI*
Octocrylene *SS*
Octoxynol 16 *ES*
Octoxynol 30 *ES*
Octoxynol 40 *ES*
Octoxynol–1 *ES*
Octoxynol–2 *DS*
Octoxynol–3 *ES*
Octoxynol–5 *ES*
Octoxynol–8 *ES WA*
Octoxynol–10 *DS ES SF*
Octoxynol–12 *SF*
Octoxynol–16 *DS*
Octoxynol–30 *DS*
Octoxynol–40 *DS*
Octoxynol–70 *DS WA*
Octrizole *SS*
Octyl benzoate *PL SO*

Octyl cocoate *EL*
Octyl decanol *EL*
Octyl dimethyl PABA *SS SS*
Octyl dodecanol *EL ES*
Octyl dodecyl behenate *EL*
Octyl hydroxystearate *EL*
Octyl isononanoate *EL*
Octyl laurate *PL SO*
Octyl methoxycinnamate *SS*
Octyl neopentanoate *EL*
Octyl octanoate *EL*
Octyl oleate *EL*
Octyl palmitate *EL SO*
Octyl pelargonate *EL*
Octyl salicylate *SS*
Octyl stearate *EL*
Octyl triazone *S*
Octylacrylamide-acrylates-butylaminoethyl methacrylate polymer *RS*
Octyldodeceth–5 *DS*
Octyldodeceth–10 *SF*
Octyldodeceth–16 *SF*
Octyldodeceth–20 *ES*
Octyldodeceth–25 *ES*
Octylodecyl benzoate *EL FA*
Octyldodecyl erucate *EL*
Octyldodecyl lactate *GL SO*
Octyldodeyl myristate *EL*
Octyldodecyl stearate *EL*
Octyldodecyl stearoyl stearate *EL*
Ointment base *EL*
Oleamide *SB TK*
Oleamide DEA *ES FA TK*
Oleamide MEA *FA TK*
Oleamide MIPA *FA*
Oleamine *CO*
Oleamine oxide *CO EL*
Oleastearine *EL*
Oleic acid *ES*
Oleic alcohol *EL*
Oleic-palmitoleic-linoleic glycerides *EL*
Oleoamphohydroxypropyl sulfonate *DT*
Oleostearine *LU*
Oleoyl diethanolamide *ES*
Oleoyl sarcosine *CO SF*

Oleth–2 *ES*
Oleth–2 phosphate *ES SF*
Oleth–3 *ES*
Oleth–3 phosphate *ES GE*
Oleth–4 *ES*
Oleth–5 *ES*
Oleth–5 phosphate *ES SF*
Oleth–6 *ES*
Oleth–7 *ES*
Oleth–8 *ES*
Oleth–9 *ES*
Oleth–10 *ES*
Oleth–10 phosphate *ES GE*
Oleth–12 *DT ES*
Oleth–13 *ES*
Oleth–15 *DT ES*
Oleth–20 *ES*
Oleth–23 *ES*
Oleth–25 *ES*
Oleth–30 *ES*
Oleth–40 *DS ES*
Oleth–50 *ES*
Oleyl alcohol *CA DS EL*
Oleyl betaine *CO FA*
Oleyl dimethylamidopropyl ethonium ethosulfate *CO*
Oleyl erucate *EL*
Oleyl hydroxyethyl imidazoline *SF*
Oleyl oleate *EL*
Olive extract *BO*
Olive leaf extract *BO*
Olive oil *EL*
Olive oil PEG–6 esters *SO*
Onion extract (Allium cepa) *BO*
Ophiopogon japonicus extract *MO*
Orange flower extract *BO*
Orange peel extract *AD BO*
Orange roughy oil *EL*
Orange wax *EL MO*
Oryzanol *AO SS*
Ouricury wax *WX*
Oxyquinline sulfate *AP*
Ozokerite *WX*

p-Chloro-m-cresol *AP*
p-Hydroxyanisole *AO*

PABA *SS*
Palm acid *ES*
Palm kernel amide DEA
  FA
Palm kernel glycerides *EL*
Palm kernel oil *VA*
Palm oil *EL*
Palmetto extract *A AD MO*
Palmitamide MEA *FA PE
  TK*
Palmitamidopropyl
  betaine *CO DT*
Palmitamidopropyl
  dimethylamine *CO ES*
Palmitamine *CO*
Palmitamine oxide *CO SF*
Palmitic acid *EL ES*
Palmitoyl collagen amino
  acids *AD*
Palmitoyl hydrolyzed milk
  protein *AD*
Palmitoyl hydrolyzed
  wheat protein *AD*
Palmitoyl keratin amino
  acids *AD*
Palmityl betaine *SF*
Pansy extract *BO SS*
Pantethine *MO*
Panethenol *HU*
Panthenyl ethyl ether *HU*
Paraffin *MO*
Parsley extract *BO*
Partially hydrogenated
  canola oil *EL*
Partially hydrogenated
  soybean oil *EL*
Passion flower extract
  (Passiflora incarnata)
  BO
PCA *HU*
PCA ethyl cocoyl arginate
  SF
Pea extract *BO*
Peach kernel oil *VA*
Peach leaf extract (Prusus
  persica) *BO*
Peanut oil *EL*
Peanut oil PEG–6 esters
  SO
Pearlescent pigments *PE*
Pectin *TK*
PEG dioleate *ES*
PEG lauryl ether sulfate *FA*

PEG–2 cocamine *AS ES*
PEG–2 cocomonium
  chloride *AS*
PEG–2 Diisononanoate *EL*
PEG–2 dioctanoate *EL*
PEG–2 distearate *OP*
PEG–2 laurate *ES TK*
PEG–2 milk solids *EL*
PEG–2 oleammonium
  chloride *AS CO*
PEG–2 oleate *ES*
PEG–2 oleyl amine *ES*
PEG–2 soyamine *ES*
PEG–2 stearamine *ES*
PEG–2 stearate *ES LU OP*
PEG–2 stearate SE *ES OP*
PEG–2 stearmonium
  chloride *CO*
PEG–2 tallow amine *ES*
PEG–3 C12-C18 alcohols
  ES
PEG–3 cocamide *ES*
PEG–3 distearate *OP PE
  TK*
PEG–3 glyceryl isostearate
  ES
PEG–3 glyceryl
  triisostearate *ES*
PEG–3 glyceryl tristearate
  ES
PEG–3 lanolate *ES*
PEG–3 lauramide *FA TK*
PEG–3 lauramine oxide
  CO FA TK
PEG–3 sorbitan oleate *ES*
PEG–3 stearate *ES RA*
PEG–4 *EL MO HU*
PEG–4 diheptanoate *EL*
PEG–4 diisostearate *ES TK*
PEG–4 dilaurate *EL LU*
PEG–4 dioleate *ES*
PEG–4 distearate *ES*
PEG–4 glyceryl distearate
  ES
PEG–4 laurate *ES*
PEG–4 oleamide *FA RA
  TK*
PEG–4 oleate *ES*
PEG–4 stearate *ES*
PEG–4 stearyl stearate *ES*
PEG–4 tallate *ES*
PEG–5 C12-C18 alcohols
  ES

PEG–5 C14–18 alcohols
  citrate *EL*
PEG–5 C8–12 alcohols
  citrate *EL*
PEG–5 castor oil *ES*
PEG–5 cocamine *ES*
PEG–5 glyceryl isostearate
  ES
PEG–5 glyceryl
  sesquioleate *DS ES*
PEG–5 glyceryl stearate *ES*
PEG–5 glyceryl
  triisostearate *ES*
PEG–5 hydrogenated
  castor oil *EL*
PEG–5 hydrogenated
  castor oil triisostearate
  EL
PEG–5 lanolate *ES*
PEG–5 oleamine *ES*
PEG–5 soya sterol *ES*
PEG–5 soyamine *ES*
PEG–5 stearamine *ES*
PEG–5 stearate *ES*
PEG–5 stearyl ammonium
  lactate *CO*
PEG–5 tallow amide *ES*
PEG–5 tallow amine *ES*
PEG–6 *EL MO*
PEG–6 beeswax *DS TK*
PEG–6 caprylic-capric
  glycerides *ES RA*
PEG–6 cocamide *ES*
PEG–6 dilaurate *ES*
PEG–6 dioleate *ES*
PEG–6 distearate *ES*
PEG–6 isostearate *ES*
PEG–6 lauramide *ES*
PEG–6 laurate *ES*
PEG–6 methyl ether *SO*
PEG–6 oleate *ES*
PEG–6 palmitate *ES*
PEG–6 paraffinic ether
  12–14 *ES*
PEG–6 sorbitan beeswax
  ES
PEG–6 sorbitan
  monolaurate *ES*
PEG–6 sorbitan
  monostearate *ES*
PEG–6 sorbitan oleate *ES*
PEG–6 undecylenate *AD*
PEG–6–32 *ES*

PEG–6–32 stearate *ES*
PEG–7 glyceryl cocoate *ES RA*
PEG–7 hydrogenated castor oil *ES*
PEG–7 oleate *ES*
PEG–7.5 tallowmine *ES*
PEG–7M *CO FA*
PEG–8 *EL ES MO HU TK*
PEG–8 beeswax *ES*
PEG–8 caprylic-capric glycerides *AS SF*
PEG–8 castor oil *ES*
PEG–8 dilaurate *EL ES*
PEG–8 dioleate *EL ES TK*
PEG–8 distearate *ES TK*
PEG–8 glyceryl laurate *ES*
PEG–8 laurate *ES SF*
PEG–8 oleate *ES*
PEG–8 paraffinic ether 12–14 *ES*
PEG–8 stearate *ES TK*
PEG–8 tallate *ES*
PEG–9 castor oil *ES*
PEG–9 diisostearate *ES*
PEG–9 dioleate *ES*
PEG–9 distearate *ES*
PEG–9 laurate *ES*
PEG–9 oleate *DS ES*
PEG–9 stearate *DS ES*
PEG–9 stearyl stearate *EL*
PEG–10 C12-C18 alcohol *ES*
PEG–10 castor oil *ES*
PEG–10 cocamine *AS ES*
PEG–10 coconut oil *ES*
PEG–10 dioleate *DS ES*
PEG–10 glyceryl isostearate *ES*
PEG–10 glyceryl stearate *DT*
PEG–10 hydrogenated castor oil triisostearate *ES*
PEG–10 lanolate *ES*
PEG–10 polyglyceryl–2 laurate *ES*
PEG–10 sorbitan laurate *ES*
PEG–10 soya sterol *ES*
PEG–10 stearamine *DS ES*
PEG–10 stearate *ES*
PEG–10 stearyl stearate *EL*

PEG–11 babassu glycerides *ES*
PEG–11 castor oil *ES*
PEG–12 *EL MO SO*
PEG–12 beeswax *DS TK*
PEG–12 dilaurate *ES*
PEG–12 dioleate *EL ES*
PEG–12 distearate *ES*
PEG–12 glyceryl dioleate *DS ES*
PEG–12 laurate *DS ES*
PEG–12 oleate *ES*
PEG–12 palm kernel glycerides *AD EL*
PEG–12 stearate *ES*
PEG–12 tallate *ES*
PEG–14 avocado glycerides *ES*
PEG–15 cocamine phosphate oleate *EL*
PEG–15 coco polyamine *CO*
PEG–15 cocomine *ES*
PEG–15 cocomonium chloride *CO*
PEG–15 glyceryl isostearate *ES*
PEG–15 glyceryl laurate *ES*
PEG–15 glyceryl ricinoleate *ES*
PEG–15 glyceryl stearate *DT SF*
PEG–15 oleamine *ES*
PEG–15 oleate *ES*
PEG–15 soyamine *AS ES*
PEG–15 stearamine *ES*
PEG–15 tallow amine *ES*
PEG–15 tallow polyamine *ES*
PEG–16 *ES RA*
PEG–16 hydrogenated castor oil *ES*
PEG–16 soya sterol *ES*
PEG–18 *EL*
PEG–18 glyceryl oleate-cocoate *TK*
PEG–18 stearate *ES*
PEG–20 *EL*
PEG–20 almond glycerides *ES RA*
PEG–20 castor oil *ES*
PEG–20 dilaurate *ES*

PEG–20 dioleate *ES*
PEG–20 distearate *ES*
PEG–20 glyceryl isostearate *DS*
PEG–20 glyceryl laurate *ES*
PEG–20 glyceryl oleate *ES*
PEG–20 glyceryl stearate *ES*
PEG–20 glyceryl triisostearate *ES*
PEG–20 glyceryl tristearate *ES*
PEG–20 hydrogenated castor oil *ES SO*
PEG–20 hydrogenated castor oil isostearate *EL*
PEG–20 hydrogenated castor oil triisostearate *EL*
PEG–20 hydrogenated lanolin *EL ES*
PEG–20 lanolin *ES*
PEG–20 laurate *ES*
PEG–20 maize glycerides *ES RA*
PEG–20 methyl glucose sesquistearate *ES*
PEG–20 oleate *ES*
PEG–20 sorbitan beeswax *ES*
PEG–20 sorbitan isostearate *ES*
PEG–20 sorbitan trioleate *ES*
PEG–20 stearate *ES*
PEG–20 tallow amine *ES*
PEG–23 oleate *ES*
PEG–23 stearate *ES*
PEG–24 hydrogenated lanolin *EL ES*
PEG–25 castor oil *DS ES*
PEG–25 glyceryl isostearate *DT SF*
PEG–25 PABA *EL SS*
PEG–25 propylene glycol stearate *EL ES*
PEG–25 soya sterol *ES*
PEG–25 stearate *ES*
PEG–27 lanolin *CO LU SF*
PEG–28 glyceryl tallowate *AD TK*

PEG–29 castor oil *ES*
PEG–30 castor oil *ES*
PEG–30 glyceryl isostearate *ES*
PEG–30 glyceryl laurate *ES*
PEG–30 glyceryl monococoate *AD*
PEG–30 glyceryl oleate *ES*
PEG–30 glyceryl stearate *ES*
PEG–30 hydrogenated castor oil *ES*
PEG–30 lanolin *ES LU SF*
PEG–30 sorbitan tetraoleate *ES*
PEG–32 dilaurate *ES*
PEG–32 dioleate *ES*
PEG–32 distearate *ES*
PEG–32 laurate *ES*
PEG–32 oleate *ES*
PEG–32 stearate *ES*
PEG–33 castor oil *SO*
PEG–35 stearate *ES*
PEG–40 castor oil *ES*
PEG–40 dodecyl glycol copolymer *ES SB*
PEG–40 glyceryl isostearate *ES*
PEG–40 glyceryl stearate *SF*
PEG–40 glyceryl triisostearate *ES*
PEG–40 hydrogenated castor oil PCA isostearate *DS*
PEG–40 hydrogenated castor oil *ES*
PEG–40 hydrogenated castor oil isostearate *EL*
PEG–40 hydrogenated castor oil laurate *EL*
PEG–40 hydrogenated castor oil PCA isostearate *ES*
PEG–40 hydrogenated castor oil triisostearate *EL*
PEG–40 jojoba oil *EL SF TK*
PEG–40 lanolin *CO LU SF*
PEG–40 sorbitan lanolate *ES*

PEG–40 sorbitan tetraoleate *ES*
PEG–40 stearate *ES LU SB*
PEG–42 babassu glycerides *ES*
PEG–44 sorbitan laurate *ES*
PEG–45 palm kernel glycerides *ES WA*
PEG–45 safflower oil glycerides
PEG–50 glyceryl cocoate *SO*
PEG–50 hydrogenated castor oil laurate *EL*
PEG–50 lanolin *ES*
PEG–50 stearmine *ES*
PEG–50 stearate *ES*
PEG–50 tallow amide *TK*
PEG–55 propylene glycol oleate *TK*
PEG–60 almond glycerides *ES WA*
PEG–60 castor oil *ES*
PEG–60 glyceryl isostearate *SF*
PEG–60 glyceryl stearate *SF*
PEG–60 glyceryl triisostearate *ES*
PEG–60 hydrogenated castor oil *ES*
PEG–60 hydrogenated castor oil isostearate *ES*
PEG–60 hydrogenated castor oil triisostearate *ES*
PEG–60 lanolin *ES*
PEG–60 maize glycerides *ES WA*
PEG–60 sorbitan tetraoleate *ES*
PEG–70 mango seed glycerides *EL ES*
PEG–75 *EL ES*
PEG–75 castor oil *ES*
PEG–75 dilaurate *ES*
PEG–75 dioleate *ES*
PEG–75 distearate *ES*
PEG–75 illipe butter glycerides *EL ES*
PEG–75 lanolin *CO EL ES*

PEG–75 lanolin oil *CO SF*
PEG–75 laurate *ES*
PEG–75 oleate *ES*
PEG–75 shea butter glycerides *EL ES*
PEG–75 stearate *ES TK*
PEG–78 glyceryl cocoate *AD*
PEG–80 jojoba oil *SF*
PEG–80 sorbitan laurate *ES FA*
PEG–82 glyceryl tallowate *AD*
PEG–85 lanolin *CO*
PEG–90 stearate *ES*
PEG–100 castor oil *ES*
PEG–100 hydrogenated castor oil *ES*
PEG–100 lanolin *ES*
PEG–100 stearate *ES MO TK*
PEG–120 distearate *ES*
PEG–120 jojoba oil *SF*
PEG–120 methyl glucose dioleate *TK*
PEG–150 *EL*
PEG–150 dilaurate *ES*
PEG–150 dioleate *ES*
PEG–150 distearate *ES TK*
PEG–150 lanolin *ES*
PEG–150 laurate *ES*
PEG–150 oleate *ES*
PEG–150 stearate *ES*
PEG–200 castor oil *ES*
PEG–200 glyceryl monotallowate *AD TK*
PEG–200 glyceryl stearate *ES TK*
PEG–200 hydrogenated castor oil *ES*
PEG–200 laurate *ES*
PEG–200 oleate *ES*
PEG–400 laurate *ES*
PEG–6000 distearate *TK*
PEG–6000 laurate *ES*
PEG-PPG–17–6 copolymer *EL LU*
Pelargonium extract *BO*
Pellitory extract *BO*
Pennyroyal extract *BO*
Pentaerythritol dioleate *EL*
Pentaerythritol stearate *EL*

Pentaerythritol
tetrabenzoate *PL*
Pentaerythritol
tetracaprylatecaprate
EL
Pentaerythritol
tetracaprylatetetra-
caprate *EL*
Pentaerythritol
tetraisononanoate *EL*
Pentaerythritol
tetraisostearate *EL*
Pentaerythritol
tetralaurate *EL*
Pentaerythritol
tetraoctanoate *EL*
Pentaerythritol tetraoleate
EL
Pentaerythritol
tetrapelagonate *EL LU*
Pentaerythritol
tetrastearate *EL*
Pentaerythrytol
tetrabehenate *TK*
Pentaerythrytol
tetracaprylatecaprate
ES
Pentaerythrytol
tetrastearate *TK*
Pentasodium pentetate
AO CH PR
Pentasodium triphosphate
SA
Pentetic acid *AO CH PR*
Peony extract *BO*
Peppermint extract
(Mentha piperita L.)
AD BO
Peppermint oil *BO*
Perfluoropolymethyl-
isopropyl ether *MO*
SB
Perilla extract *BO*
Periwinkle extract *BO*
Petrolatum *EL MO LU*
Petroleum distillates *SO*
Petroleum wax *MO*
Phenethyl alcohol *PR*
Phenoxyethanol *AD*
Phenoxyisopropanol *AD*
Phenyl dimethicone *EL*
Phenyl trimethicone *CO*
EL GL

Phenylmercuric acetate
AD
Phenylmercuric benzoate
AD
Phenylmercuric borate *AD*
Phenylmethylpolysilox-
anes *EL*
Philodendron extract *AD*
Phosphate esters *ES*
Phosphated amine oxides
ES
Phytic acid *CH*
Pimento extract *BO*
Pine cone extract (Pinus
silvestris L.) *BO*
Pine needle extract *BO*
Pineapple extract *BO*
Piroctone olamine *AD*
Pistachio nut oil *EL MO*
Placental enzymes *EL*
Placental protein, water
soluble *MO*
Plankton extract *MO*
Plantain extract (Plantago
lanceolata) *BO*
Ploysorbate *DS*
POE–25 phytostanol *ES*
POE–30 sorbitol
tetraoleate *ES*
POE–60 sorbitol
tetraoleate *ES*
Pollen extract *BO*
Poloamer 105 benzoate *EL*
Poloxamer 101 *DS ES SF*
Poloxamer 105 *ES GE TK*
Poloxamer 122 *DS ES SF*
Poloxamer 123 *ES GE WA*
Poloxamer 124 *ES GE TK*
Poloxamer 181 *DS ES WA*
Poloxamer 182 *DS ES WA*
Poloxamer 182 dibenzoate
EL
Poloxamer 184 *DS ES WA*
Poloxamer 185 *ES GE TK*
Poloxamer 235 *ES GE WA*
Poloxamer 237 *ES GE TK*
Poloxamer 238 *ES GE TK*
Poloxamer 334 *ES WA*
Poloxamer 338 *ES GE TK*
Poloxamer 407 *ES GE TK*
Poly oxyethylene
(dimethylamino)
ethylene dichloride *PR*

Polyacrylamidomethylpro-
pane sulfonic acid *LU*
Polyacrylic acid *TK*
Polyamino sugar
condensate *MO HU*
Polyaminopropyl
biguanide *PR*
Polybutane *LU*
Polybutene *EL MO*
Polydecene *EL*
Polyethylene, ionomer *FF*
Polyethylene,
homopolymer *GE SA*
Polyethylene, micronized
SA
Polyethylene, oxidized *GE*
Polyethylene glycol *EL*
Polyethylenepaste *SB*
Polyglycerol–10 tetra
oleate *EL ES*
Polyglyceryl methacrylate
MO LU
Polyglyceryl–2
diisostearate *EL*
Polyglyceryl–2 dioleate *ES*
Polyglyceryl–2 isostearate
ES
Polyglyceryl–2 oleate *ES*
Polyglyceryl–2 PEG–4
stearate *ES*
Polyglyceryl–2 stearate *ES*
Polyglyceryl–2
tetraisostearate *EL*
Polyglyceryl–2
triisostearate *EL*
Polyglyceryl–3 beeswax
WX
Polyglyceryl–3
diisostearate *DS EL SF*
SO
Polyglyceryl–3 dioleate *ES*
Polyglyceryl–3 distearate
EL ES
Polyglyceryl–3 methyl
glucose distearate *ES*
Polyglyceryl–3 oleate *ES*
Polyglyceryl–3 stearate *EL*
ES
Polyglyceryl–4 oleate *ES*
Polyglyceryl–4 stearate *ES*
Polyglyceryl–5 distearate
DS
Polyglyceryl–6 dioleate *ES*

Polyglyceryl–6 distearate *ES*

Polyglyceryl–6 laurate *ES*

Polyglyceryl–6 mixed fatty acid *DS*

Polyglyceryl–6 myristate *ES*

Polyglyceryl–6 oleate *ES*

Polyglyceryl–6 polyricinoleate *ES*

Polyglyceryl–6 stearate *ES*

Polyglyceryl–8 oleate *ES*

Polyglyceryl–10 decaoleate *EL ES*

Polyglyceryl–10 decastearate *EL*

Polyglyceryl–10 diisostearate *ES*

Polyglyceryl–10 diistearate *DS*

Polyglyceryl–10 dioleate *ES*

Polyglyceryl–10 dipalmitate *ES*

Polyglyceryl–10 distearate *DS ES*

Polyglyceryl–10 laurate *ES*

Polyglyceryl–10 linoleate *ES*

Polyglyceryl–10 mixed fatty acids *ES*

Polyglyceryl–10 myristate *ES*

Polyglyceryl–10 oleate *ES*

Polyglyceryl–10 sostearate *ES*

Polyglyceryl–10 stearate *ES*

Polyglyceryl–10 tetraoleate *ES*

Polyglyceryl–10 trioleate *ES*

Polyisobutene (hyd.) *EL*

Polyisobutene / isohexopentacentahectane *EL GL*

Polyisobutene / isooctahexacontane *EL GL*

Polyisobutene / isopentacontaoctane *EL*

Polyisoprene *EL*

Polymethacrylamidopropyl trimonium chloride *CO*

Polymethoxy bicyclic oxazolidine *PR*

Polyoxyethylene dihydroxy-propyl linoleaminium chloride *CO*

Polyoxyethylene glycol dibenzoate *SO PL*

Poloxyethylene polyoxypropylene *ES*

Polyoxyethylene polyoxypropylene glycol *EL*

Polyoxyethylene–15 cocamine phospaheoleate complex *EL*

Polypropylene *RS*

Polypropylene glycol dibenzoate *SO PL*

Polyquaternium–2 *EL CO*

Polyquaternium–5 *ES CO*

Polyquaternium–6 *CO*

Polyquaternium–7 *CO*

Polyquaternium–10 *ES FX*

Polyquaternium–11 *CO*

Polyquaternium–16 *CO RS*

Polyquaternium–17 *CO*

Polyquaternium–18 *CO*

Polyquaternium–22 *CO*

Polyquaternium–24 *CO*

Polyquaternium–29 *FX CO*

Polyquaternium–31 *GE*

Polyquaternium–39 *CO*

Polysiloxane polyalkylene copolymer *EL*

Polysiloxane-polyether copolymer *SF*

Polysorbate 20 *ES TK*

Polysorbate 21 *ES*

Polysorbate 40 *EL ES*

Polysorbate 60 *ES WA*

Polysorbate 61 *ES*

Polysorbate 65 *ES*

Polysorbate 80 *ES WA*

Polysorbate 81 *ES*

Polysorbate 85 *ES*

Polytrimonium hydrolyzed animal protein *AD*

Polyvinyl acetate *FF*

Polyvinyl alcohol *FF*

Potassium abietoyl hydrolyzed collagen *AP PT*

Potassium alginate *GE*

Potassium aspartate *CH*

Potassium cetyl phosphate *ES*

Potassium chloride *TK*

Potassium cocoyl hydrolyzed collagen *DT PT SF*

Potassium dimethicone copolyol panethenyl phosphate *CO*

Potassium dimethicone copolyol phosphate *EL*

Potassium DNA *MO*

Potassium laurate *ES LU*

Potassium lauroyl collagen amino acids *CO*

Potassium lauroyl hydrolyzed collagen *SF*

Potassium lauroyl hydrolyzed soybean protein *CO*

Potassium lauroyl wheat amino acids *CO*

Potassium lauryl sulfate *FA SF*

Potassium myristate *ES LU*

Potassium myristoyl hydrolyzed collagen *PT SF*

Potassium oleate *TK*

Potassium oleoyl hydrolyzed collagen *PT SF*

Potassium palmitate *SF*

Potassium PCA *MO*

Potassium polyacrylate *DS*

Potassium sorbate *AD*

Potassium stearate *TK*

Potassium steroyl hydrolyzed collagen

Potassium tallowate *ES LU*

Potassium undecylenoyl hydrolyzed collagen *PT SF*

PPG–2 lanolin ether *EL*

PPG–2 myristyl ether propionate *SO EL LU*

PPG–2-buteth–3 *EL*

PPG–2-ceteareth–9 *ES*

PPG–2-isodeceth–4 *SF*
PPG–2-isodeceth–6 *SF*
PPG–2-isodeceth–9 *SF*
PPG–2-isodeceth–12 *SF*
PPG–3 hydrogenated
castor oil *EL*
PPG–3 isosteareth–9 *ES*
PPG–3 myristyl ether *EL*
LU
PPG–5 buteth–7 *ES*
PPG–5 ceteth–10
phosphate *ES*
PPG–5 lanolin ether *CO*
PPG–5 lanolin wax *EL SB*
PPG– pentaerythrityl ether
EL
PPG–5-buteth–7 *EL*
PPG–5-butyl ether *EL*
PPG–5-ceteth–20 *ES*
PPG–5-laureth–5 *EL*
PPG–6 C12–18 pareth–11
SF
PPG–7-buteth–10 *SB*
PPG–7-buteth–5 *EL*
PPG–8 oleate *ES*
PPG–8-SMDI copolymer
EL MO
PPG–9 *EL*
PPG–9 diethylmonium
chloride *AS CO*
PPG–9 Diethylmonium
phosphate *DS*
PPG–9-buteth–12 *EL LU*
PPG–9-butyl ether *EL*
PPG–10 butanediol *EL MO*
PPG–10 cetyl ether *CA EL*
PPG–10 cetyl ether
phosphate *ES SB*
PPG–10 lanolin alcohol
ether *WA*
PPG–10 methyl glucose
ether *EL GL*
PPG–10 oleyl ether *CA EL*
PPG–11 stearyl ether *EL*
LU
PPG–12 PEG–65 lanolin
oil *EL*
PPG–12-buteth–16 *EL LU*
PPG–12-PEG–50 lanolin
EL ES LU
PPG–12 / SMDI
copolymer *EL MO*
PPG–14 butyl ether *EL LU*

PPG–15 butyl ether *EL*
PPG–15 stearyl ether *CA EL*
PPG–15 stearyl ether
benzoate *EL FA*
PPG–16 butyl ether *EL*
PPG–18 butyl ether *EL*
PPG–20 *EL*
PPG–20 lanolin alcohol
ether *PL SO CO*
PPG–20 methyl glucose
ether *FX*
PPG–20 methyl glucose
ether distearate *MO*
PPG–20-buteth–30 *EL LU*
PPG–22 butyl ether *CA*
PPG–23 oleyl ether *CA*
PPG–24-buteth–27 *ES LU*
PPG–24-glycereth–24
polyglycol copolymer
EL
PPG–25 Diethylmonium
chloride *AS DS*
PPG–25 laureth–25 *ES*
PPG–26 *EL*
PPG–26 oleate *ES*
PPG–26-buteth–26 *ES*
PPG–27 glyceryl ether *EL*
PPG–28-buteth–30 *EL*
PPG–28-buteth–35 *LU*
PPG–30 *EL*
PPG–30 cetyl ether *EL*
PPG–36 oleate *ES GL LU*
PPG–40 butyl ether *EL LU*
PPG–40 Diethylmonium
chloride *AS DS*
PPG–50 cetyl ether *EL*
PPG–50 oleyl ether *CA EL*
PPG–51-SMDI copolymer
EL MO
PPG–53 butyl ether *EL*
Procollagen *FF*
Proline *CO*
Propane *PP*
Propionyl collagen amino
acids *AD*
Propyl alcohol *SO*
Propyl gallate *AO*
Propylene carbonate *SB*
Propylene glycol *SO*
Propylene glycol ceteth–3
acetate *EL*
Propylene glycol
dibenzoate *PL SO*

Propylene glycol
dicaprylate *EL*
Propylene glycol
dicaprylate-dicaprate
EL
Propylene glycol
diisostearate *EL*
Propylene glycol dioleate
ES
Propylene glycol
dipelargonate *EL RA*
Propylene glycol distearate
ES OP
Propylene glycol
dioctanoate *EL*
Propylene glycol
hydroxystearate *ES*
Propylene glycol
isoceteth–3 acetate
EL
Propylene glycol
isostearate *EL*
Propylene glycol laurate
EL ES
Propylene glycol methyl
ether *SO*
Propylene glycol myristate
EL OP
Propylene glycol myristate
SO
Propylene glycol myristyl
ether acetate *EL PL*
Propylene glycol
ricinoleate *ES*
Propylene glycol stearate,
SE *EL ES*
Propylene glycol stearate
AS CO ES OP TK
Propylparaben *PR*
Propyltrimonium
hydrolyzed wheat
protein *PT*
Proteoglycan, soluble *CO*
PT
PVM / MA decadiene
crosspolymer *TK*
PVP *RS TK*
PVP-Dimethiconylacrylate-
polycarbamyl-
polyglycol ester *FF CO*
PVP-dimethylaminoethyl
methacrylate
copolymer *CO*

PVP-eicosene copolymer *DS FF*
PVP-hexadecene copolymer *DS FF*
PVP-iodine *AP*
PVP / dimethylaminoethyl methacrylate polycarbamyl polyglycol ester *CO FF*
Pyridoxine HCL *VT*

Quaternium–15 *PR*
Quaternium–18 bentonite *SA TK*
Quaternium–18 hectorite *SA TK*
Quaternium–22 *CO HU*
Quaternium–26 *AS CO*
Quaternium–27 *AS*
Quaternium–33 *CO ES*
Quaternium–53 *AS*
Quaternium–61 *CO*
Quaternium–62 *AS CO*
Quaternium–70 *AS CO*
Quaternium–72 *AS CO*
Quaternium–73 *AD*
Quaternium–76 hydrolyzed collagen *CO*
Quaternium–79 hydrolyzed keratin *LU PT*
Quaternium–79 hydrolyzed silk *LU PT*
Quaternium–80 *CO SI*
Queen of the meadow extract *BO*
Quillaja extract (Quillaja saponaria. Mol.) *SF FA*
Quince seed extract *BO*

Raffinose laurate *SF*
Raffinose myristate *SF*
Raffinose oleate *SF*
Raffinose palmitate *SF*
Raffinose stearate *SF*
Rapeseed amidopropyl benzyldimonium chloride Quarternium–61 *CO*
Rapeseed amidopropyl epoxypropyl dimonium chloride *CO*

Rapeseed amidopropyl ethyldimonium ethosulfate *CO ES*
Rapeseed oil, ethoxylated high erucic acid *DS TK*
Rapeseed oil *EL*
Rapeseed amido-propyl benzyldimonium chloride *AS*
Rapeseed amidopropyl epoxypropyl dimonium chloride *AS*
Rauwolfia extract *BO*
Rehmannia root extract *MO*
Resorcinol *AD*
Restharrow extract *BO*
Rhododenron extract *BO*
Rhubarb extract *BO*
Riboflavin tetraacetate *VT*
Ribonucleic acid *PT*
Rice bran extract *BO*
Rice bran oil *EL MO VA*
Rice bran wax *ES PL*
Rice germ oil *HU*
Rice peptide *CO FF PT*
Rice starch *LU*
Ricinoleamide DEA *ES*
Ricinoleamide MEA *FA TK*
Ricinoleamidopropyl betaine *CO SF*
Ricinoleamidopropyl dimethylamine lactate *CO*
Ricinoleamidopropyl ethyldimonium ethosulfate *CO*
Ricinoleamidopropyl trimethyl ammonium ethosulfate *CO*
Ricinoleamidopropyl-dimonium ethosulfate *CO*
Ricinoleamidopropyl-trimonium chloride *CO*
Ricinoleamidopropyl trimethyl ammononium ethosulfate *AD*
Ricinoleic acid *ES*
Ricinoleyl alcohol *DS*
Rose extract (Rosa spp.) *BO*

Rose hips extract *BO*
Rose hips oil *EL*
Rose seed extract *MO*
Rosemary extract (Rosmarinus officinalis) *BO*
Royal jelly extract *MO*

Saccharide isomerate *MO*
Safflower extract *BO*
Safflower oil *EL*
Sage extract (Salvia officinalis L.) *BO*
Salmon egg extract *EL*
Sambucus extract *BO*
Sandalwood extract *BO*
Sanguinaria root extract *BO*
Sanguisorbae radix extract *A*
Saponaria extract (Saponaria officinalis L.) *BO*
Saponins *ES*
Saxifraga sarmentosa extract *BO*
Scabiosae extract *BO*
Scutellaria root extract *BO*
Sea bottom *BO*
Sea buckthorn oil *VA*
Sea Salts *HU*
Selenium aspartate *MO*
Selenium protein complex *ES MO*
Serum albumin *MO PT*
Sesame oil *EL*
Sesamide DEA *FA TK*
Shark liver oil *EL*
Shea butter *EL*
Shellac *FF*
Shikonin *AP*
Silica, colloidal *AS*
Silicone quaternium–3 *CO*
Silicone quaternium–4 *CO*
Silicone quaternium–5 *ES*
Silicone quaternium–6 *ES*
Silk amino acids *CO MO*
Silk powder *PT*
Sitostearyl acetate *EL*
Skin lipids *EL*
Sodium alpha olefin sulfonate *SF*

Sodium aluminium
chlorohydroxy lactate
DO
Sodium ascorbate *AO*
Sodium aspartate *CH*
Sodium behenoyl lactylate
HU
Sodium benzoate *PR*
Sodium butoxyethoxy
acetate *WA*
Sodium C8–16
isoalkylsuccinyl
lactoglobulin sulfonate
EL
Sodium C12–13 sulfate *SF*
Sodium C12–14 pareth–2
sulfate *SF*
Sodium C12–15 pareth–3
sulfonate *FA SF*
Sodium C12–15 pareth–7
carboxylate *SF*
Sodium C12–15 pareth–7
sulfonate *FF SF*
Sodium C12–15 pareth–8
carboxylate *SF*
Sodium C12–15 pareth–15
sulfonate *ES FA SF AD*
Sodium C12–15 pareth
sulfate *SF*
Sodium C12–18 alkyl
sulfate *SF*
Sodium C13-C17 alkane
sulfonate *SF*
Sodium C14–16 olefin
sulfonate *SF*
Sodium C14–17 alkyl
sulfonate *DT*
Sodium
caproamphoacetate *DT*
Sodium
caproamphohydroxy-
propylsulfonate *FA*
Sodium caproyl lactylate
ES HU
Sodium
capryloamohohydroxy
propylsulfonate *WA*
Sodium carbomer *TK*
Sodium carrageenan *TK*
Sodium caseinate *PT*
Sodium cetearyl sulfate *SF*
Sodium cetyl oleyl sulfate
SF

Sodium cetyl sulfate *ES*
Sodium chloride *CR TK*
Sodium chondroitin
sulfate *MO*
Sodium citrate *BF CO*
Sodium coco hydrolyzed
collagen *PT SF*
Sodium coco-hydrolyzed
soy protein *DT PT*
Sodium coco-tallow sulfate
SF
Sodium
cocoamphoacetate *DT*
FA
Sodium
cocoamphopropionate
FA DT
Sodium
cocomonoglyceride
sulfate *DT*
Sodium cocoyl glutamate
SF
Sodium cocoyl hydrolyzed
collagen *PT SF*
Sodium cocoyl hydrolyzed
soy protein *CO*
Sodium cocoyl isethionate
DT SF
Sodium cocoyl lactylate *HU*
Sodium cocoyl sarcosinate
SF
Sodium deceth sulfate *DT*
FA
Sodium decyl diphenyl
ether sulfonate *DT WA*
Sodium dehydroacetate
PR
Sodium DNA *MO*
Sodium dodecylbenzene
sulfonate *DT*
Sodium dodecyldiphenyl
ether sulfonate *DT WA*
Sodium erythorbate *AO*
Sodium glyceryl oleate
phosphate *EL*
Sodium
hexametaphosphate
CH
Sodium hyaluronate *EL FF*
HU
Sodium hydrogenated
tallow dimethyl
glycinate *CO*

Sodium hydrogenated
tallow glutamate *SF*
Sodium
hydroxymethylglyc-
inate *PR*
Sodium iodate *DT*
Sodium isodecyl sulfate *SF*
Sodium isostearoyl
lactylate *ES HU*
Sodium lactate *HU*
Sodium laureth sulfate *DT*
SF
Sodium laureth–1 sulfate
DT FA
Sodium laureth–2 sulfate
DT FA
Sodium laureth–3 sulfate
DT FA
Sodium laureth–5
carboxylate *SF*
Sodium laureth–7 sulfate
DT FA
Sodium laureth–11
carboxylate *SF*
Sodium laureth–12 sulfate
DT
Sodium laureth–13
carboxylate *DT SF*
Sodium laureth–17
carboxylate *ES*
Sodium
lauriminodipropionate
DT FA
Sodium
lauroamphoacetate
SF
Sodium lauroamphoprop-
ionate *DT*
Sodium lauroyl collagen
amino acids *CO*
Sodium lauroyl glutamate
SF
Sodium lauroyl hydrolyzed
collagen *SF*
Sodium lauroyl keratin
amino acids *CO*
Sodium lauroyl lactylate
ES HU
Sodium lauroyl methyl
alaninate *DT*
Sodium lauroyl taurate *SF*
Sodium lauroyl wheat
amino acids *CO*

Sodium lauryl phosphate *DT*

Sodium lauryl sulfate *DT FA*

Sodium lauryl sulfoacetate *DT FA*

Sodium lauryl sulfosuccinate *FA*

Sodium laurylether sulfosuccinate *FA*

Sodium lignosulfonate *DS*

Sodium magnesium laureth sulfate *FA SF*

Sodium magnesium silicate *TK*

Sodium methyl cocoyl taurate *DT SF*

Sodium methyl naphthalene sulfonate *DT*

Sodium methyl oleoyltaurate *DT SF*

Sodium methylparaben *PR*

Sodium myreth sulfate *DT FA*

Sodium myristoyl glutamate *SF*

Sodium myristoyl hydrolyzed collagen *SF PT*

Sodium miristyl sulfate *DT FA SF*

Sodium N,N-Bis(2-hydroxyethyl) glycinate *CH*

Sodium N-cocoyl methyltaurate *DT*

Sodium N-lauroyl methyltaurate *DT*

Sodium nonoxynol–6 phosphate *ES GE SF*

Sodium o-phenylphenate *PR*

Sodium octyl sulfate *DT ES SF*

Sodium oleate *ES*

Sodium olefin C14–16 sulfonate *DT FA*

Sodium oleoyl hydrolyzed collagen *PT SF*

Sodium oleyl sulfate *DT ES*

Sodium pareth–25 sulfate *DT FA*

Sodium PCA *HU*

Sodium PEG–3 octyl phenol sulfonate *FF SF*

Sodium POE alkyl ether acetate *DT*

Sodium polyglutamate *HU*

Sodium polymethacrylate *DS EL*

Sodium polynaphthalene sulfonate *DS SA*

Sodium propylparaben *PR*

Sodium pyrithione *AD PR*

Sodium ricinoleate *AD*

Sodium salicylate *AP PR*

Sodium stearate *TK*

Sodium stearoamphoacetate *CO*

Sodium stearoyl hydrolyzed collagen *PT SF*

Sodium stearoyl lactylate *ES HU*

Sodium tallowate *GE*

Sodium trideceth ether sulfate *DT FA*

Sodium trideceth–7 carboxylate *DT*

Sodium tridecyl sulfate *DT FA*

Sodium tripolyphosphate *SF*

Sodium undecylenoyl hydrolyzed collagen *PT SF*

Sodium-N-cocoyl methyl taurate *SF*

Sodium-PG-propyldimethicone thiosulfate *SI*

Sodium-TEA lauroyl collagen amino acids *CO*

Sodium-TEA lauroyl keratin amino acids *CO*

Sodium / TEA-lauryl hydrolyzed keratin *SF*

Soluble collagen *FF PT*

Soluble keratin *CO FF PT*

Soluble wheat protein *CO FF PT*

Sophora japonica extract *BO*

Sorbeth–20 *EL ES*

Sorbic acid *PR*

Sorbitan caprylate *AS*

Sorbitan isostearate *EL ES*

Sorbitan laurate *ES HU SB*

Sorbitan oleate *DS ES*

Sorbitan palmitate *EL ES*

Sorbitan sesquiisostearate *ES HU TK*

Sorbitan sesquioleate *EL ES*

Sorbitan sesquistearate *EL ES*

Sorbitan stearate *ES*

Sorbitan trioleate *EL ES*

Sorbitan tristearate *ES TK*

Sorbitol *HU*

Soy ethyldimonium ethosulfate *AS CO*

Soy germ extract *BO*

Soy protein *BO PT*

Soy sterol *BO*

Soyaethyl morpholinium ethosulfate *AS CO*

Soyamide DEA *CO TK*

Soyamidopropyl benzyldimonium chloride *CO*

Soyamidopropyl betaine *CO FA TK*

Soyamidopropyl ethyldimonium ethosulfate *CO*

Soyamine *ES*

Soybean extract *BO*

Soybean oil *EL*

Soytrimonium chloride *CO*

Spearmint extract *BO*

Spearmint oil *BO*

Spermaceti *EL WX*

Spherical cellulose acetate *MO*

Sphingolipids *EL HU*

Spinach extract *BO*

Spiraea extract *BO*

Spiraea extract (Filipendula ulmaria L.) *BO*

Squalane *EL MO*

Squalene *EL*

Starch polyacrylonitrile

copolymer-potassium salt *TK*

Starch polyacrylonitrile copolymer-sodium salt *TK*

Stearalkonium bentonite *TK*

Stearalkonium chloride *AS*

Stearalkonium hectorite *SA TK*

Stearamide *OP TK*

Stearamide DEA *ES TK*

Sucrose stearate *ES*

Sulfated castor oil *SF WA*

Sunflower seed extract *BO*

Sunflower seed oil *EL VA*

Super oxide dismutase *ES MO*

Super oxide dismutase liposome *CR MO*

Sweet almond oil *EL*

Sweet cherry extract *BO*

Sweet cicely extract *BO*

Sweet clover extract *BO*

Swertia extract *BO*

Synthetic beeswax *ES GE TK*

Synthetic candelilla *WX*

Synthetic carnauba *WX*

Synthetic wax *EL*

t-Butylhydroquinone *AO*

Talc *PE*

Tallow *EL*

Tallow glyceride, acetylated hydrogenated *ES*

Tallowamide MEA *TK*

Tallowamidopropyldim-ethylamine *ES*

Talloweth-6 *ES*

Talloweth-60 myristyl glycol *TK*

Tallowmide DEA *ES*

Tallowmide MEA *FA*

Tallowmidopropyldim-ethylamine *CO*

Tannic extract *A*

Tea extract *AO*

Tea tree oil *BO*

TEA-acrylates-acrylonitrogens copolymer *ES FF GE TK*

TEA-C12–15 alkyl sulfate *SF*

TEA-cocoyl hydrolyzed collagen *PT SF*

TEA-cocoyl hydrolyzed soy protein *SF*

TEA-cocoylglutamate *SF*

TEA-dodecylbenzene-sulfonate *DT FA*

TEA-hydrogenated tallow glutamate *SF*

TEA-hydroiodide *ST*

TEA-laureth sulfate *DT FA*

TEA-lauroyl collagen amino acids *FA PT*

TEA-lauroyl glutamate *SF*

TEA-lauroyl keratin amino acids *FA PT SF*

TEA-lauroyl sarcosinate *SF*

TEA-lauryl sulfate *DT FA SF*

TEA-myristoyl hydrolyzed collagen *SF*

TEA-palm kernel sarcosinate *DT FA*

TEA-PCA *HU*

TEA-PEG–3 cocamide sulfate *DT*

TEA-salicylate *SS*

Tetradecycleicosyl stearate *EL*

Tetramethyl trihyroxy hexadecane *CO*

Tetrasodium dicarboxyethyl stearyl sulfosuccinate *ES*

Tetrasodium EDTA *AO CH PR*

Thimerosal *AD*

Thistle extract *BO*

Thyme extract (Thymus vulgaris) *BO*

Thymol *DN*

Tissue extract *ES MO*

Titanated micas *PE*

Titanium dioxide *SS*

Titanium dioxide coated mica *PE*

Tocopherol *AO*

Tocopheryl acetate *AD EL*

Tocopheryl acetate *MO*

Tocopheryl linoleate *MO*

Tocopheryl nicotinate *AD ST*

Tocopheryl succinate *VT*

Toluenesulfonamide epoxy resin *PL FF*

Tomato extract (Solanum lycopersicum L.) *MO BO*

Tormentil extract *BO*

Tragacanth gum *SA TK*

Tri-lauryl phosphate *SF*

Tri-PABA-panthenol *SS*

Tribehenin *EL GE LU TK*

Tributyl citrate *PL*

Tricaprin *EL SB*

Tricaprylin *EL*

Triceteareth–4 phosphate *ES*

Tricetylmonium chloride *CO*

Triclosan *AD*

Tricontanyl PVP *DS FF*

Tricedeth–3 *ES*

Tricedeth–5 *ES*

Tricedeth–6 *ES*

Tricedeth–7 *ES*

Tricedeth–7 carboxylic acid *SF*

Tricedeth–8 *ES*

Tricedeth–9 *ES SF*

Tricedeth–10 *ES*

Tricedeth–12 *ES*

Tricedeth–15 *ES*

Tridecyl behenate *EL*

Tridecyl cocoate *EL*

Tridecyl erucate *EL*

Tridecyl ethoxylate *ES SF*

Tridecyl neopentanoate *EL*

Tridecyl octanoate *EL*

Tridecyl salicylate *CO*

Tridecyl stearate *EL*

Tridecyl stearoyl stearate *EL*

Tridecyl trimelliate *EL*

Triethanolamine C10–14 sulfate *SF*

Triethonium hydrolyzed collagen ethosulfate *CO*

Triethyl citrate *PL*

Triheptanoate *EL*

Trihydroxystearin *SA TK*

Triisocetyl citrate *EL WA*

Triisostearin *EL*

Triisostearin PEG–6 esters DS OP WA
Triisostearyl citrate EL LU
Triisostearyl trilinoleate EL
Trilaureth–5 phosphate ES
Trilaurin EL SB
Trilinolein EL
Trimethylglycine MO
Trimethyl pentanediol dibenzoate PL
Trimethylglycine AD
Trimethylolpropane tricocoate EL
Trimethylolpropane trilaurate EL
Trimethylolpropane-tricaprylate-tricaprate EL
Trimethylsilyamodime-thicone CO
Trimonium hydroxypropyl hydrolyzed collagen CO PT
Trimystin EL SB
Trioctanoate EL SB
Trioctanoin EL
Trioctyl citrate EL
Trioctyldodecyl citrate EL
Triolein EL ES LU
Tripalmitin EL SB
Tripotassium EDTA CH
Tripropylene glycol citrate EL
Tripropylene glycol methyl ether SO
Tris(hydroxymethyl)nitro methane PR
Trisodium EDTA CH PR
Trisodium HEDTA CH PR
Tristearin EL ES SB

Triundecanoin EL
Tromethamine BF
Tromethamine magnesium aluminium silicate SA TK
Tuberose extract BO

Undecylenamide DEA AD
Undecylenamidopropyl betaine DT
Undecylenamidopropyl-trimonium methosulfate AD
Undecylenic acid AD
Undecylenoyl collagen amino acids AD
Urocanic acid ST
Usnic acid PR

Walnut extract (Junglas regia L.) BO
Walnut oil EL
Walnut shell extract BO
Watercress extract (Nasturtium officinalis R. Br.) BO
Wheat bran lipids BO
Wheat germ extract BO
Wheat germ oil EL VA
Wheat germamide DEA FA TK
Wheat germamidoprop-alkonium chloride CO
Wheat germamidopropyl betaine FA SF TK
Wheat germamidopropyl dimethylamine lactate CO
Wheat germamidopropyl

ethyl dimonium ethosulfate AS CO
Wheat peptide CO FF PT
White nettle extract (Lamium album L.) BO
White willow bark extract BO
Wild indigo BO
Wild pansy extract (Viola tricolor L.) BO
Willow bark extract AD BO
Willow leaf extract (Salix alba L.) BO
Witch hazel extract (Hamamelis virginia L.) A BO
Xanthan gum SA TK

Yarrow extract (Achilea millefolium L.) BO
Yeast extract (Saccharomyces cerevisiae) EL ST
Yeast powder, deproteinated CO
Yogurt filtrate MO
Yucca extract BO FA

Zedoary oil BO ST
Zinc aspartate MO
Zinc DNA ST
Zinc laurate PE
Zinc oxide AD SS SS
Zinc PCA AD PR
Zinc phenosulfonate DO
Zinc pryithione AD
Zinc ricinoleate DO
Zinc stearate LU
Zinc undecylenate AD

Index

Page numbers in *italics* refer to illustrations